REVIEWS FROM READERS OF PROSTATE CANCER BREAKTHROUGHS

5/5 Stars: "I cannot recommend it enough! Jay Cohen tells you everything you need to know and how to try to find out more if your PSA has gone up, and what you can do about it. The more information you have, the better. This book will really help you make a decision about what you should do if you might have prostate cancer, or do have prostate cancer." *Stan F., June 18, 2013*

5/5 Stars: "I have prostate cancer; this book describes the steps one must take to insure choosing the best treatment for prostate cancer. Wish I would have had this before starting my treatment, would have done treatments differently, I'm sure with better results." *Richard, May 28, 2013*

5/5 Stars: "This book answers all the right questions. Even the ones you don't think to ask. Every man who has had a PSA test should read this!" *Anne G., Lukeville, AZ. Aug. 23, 2013.*

5/5 Stars: "If you buy only one book on the subject or for that matter numerous ones, include this book in your selection! Dr. Cohen, himself a victim of prostate cancer, avoided a recommended radical prostatectomy by going into severe research mode and ferreting out the current state-of-the-art in prostate cancer care. This is an up-to-date and well done bit of research." *Sandy S., Seminole, FL, June 6, 2013.*

5/5 Stars: "This is a Must read book for any one with prostate cancer! Up to date, very important as many options were not around a few years ago, ie imaging etc. It is written by a doctor with prostate cancer. Written on a level most people can understand and benefit from. He writes rather like he is talking to a friend but does list specifics; tests, scans, PSA numbers etc. Reads smooth and easy. ALL men should read this book and any woman who has men in their lives also would benefit also!" *Karey L., June 12, 2013.*

5/5 Stars: "If I were going to go through the process again, I would start with Dr Cohen's book." *Positive Change, May 27, 2013.*

5/5 Stars: "The book that every man with an elevated PSA or has been recently diagnosed with prostate cancer should read. I have been on active surveillance for low grade prostate cancer for three years. My provider has been wanting me to do another biopsy because it has been two years since my last one. This book did an excellent job of helping me understand the cutting-edge state-of-the-art options that are available. It also it helped direct me to one of the leading physicians doing directed prostate biopsies by color Doppler. Prostate cancer with its many options for treatment and monitoring can be quite difficult for a patient to navigate through. This book was a needed guide to help men make the best choice for them." *James B., Sept. 8, 2013.*

5/5 Stars: "For women and the men they care about: this is a great book for women who want to know about prostate cancer so they can help husbands, boyfriends, brothers, sons, fathers and male friends they love. Extremely clear and well written, the book's 110 pages explain why getting PSA testing is so important, and how to keep the doctors from misinterpreting the results. As the book says, 85% of men diagnosed with prostate cancer get surgery or radiation, yet only 15% really need it. Prostate Cancer Breakthroughs explains how to make sure your men get the right diagnostic tests and end up with the right treatment." *Barbara, Health Care Professional, April 21, 2013.*

See more independent reviews from readers on page 173

OTHER BOOKS BY JAY S. COHEN M.D.

Over Dose: The Case Against The Drug Companies. Prescription Drugs, Side Effects, and Your Health. Tarcher/Putnam, New York: October 2001.

15 Proven-Effective Natural Remedies for Migraines Headaches in Adults and Children. Square One Publishers, New York: May 2012.

What You Need to Know about Statin Drugs and Their Natural Alternatives. Square One Publishers, New York: January 2005.

Natural Alternates to Lipitor, Zocor & Other Statin Drugs. Square One Publishers, New York: 2006.

The Magnesium Solution for High Blood Pressure. How to Use Magnesium to Help Prevent & Relieve Hypertension Naturally. Square One Publishers, New York: May 2004.

The Magnesium Solution for Migraine Headaches: How to Use Magnesium to Help Prevent & Relieve Migraine and Cluster Headaches Naturally. Square One Publishers, New York: June 2004.

Make Your Medicine Safe: How To Prevent Side Effects From The Drugs You Take. New York: Avon Books, 1998, 604 pages.

The American Garden Guidebooks: A Guide to America's Finest Gardens for the General Traveler. Volumes I & II. Everitt Miller, co-author. Evans and Company, Inc., New York. Volume I: 1987; Volume II: 1988.

PROSTATE CANCER BREAKTHROUGHS 2014

NEW TESTS, NEW TREATMENTS, BETTER OPTIONS

A STEP-BY-STEP GUIDE
TO CUTTING EDGE DIAGNOSTIC TESTS
AND 12 MEDICALLY-PROVEN TREATMENTS

Jay S. Cohen, M.D.

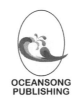

OCEANSONG
PUBLISHING

DISCLAIMER

The purpose of this book is informational and educational. The information and advice contained herein are based upon the research and the personal and professional experience of the author. This information should not be considered as a substitute for the medical advice of your health care professional. Although the information and ideas presented in this book are meant to help the reader make decisions about testing and treatment for prostate cancer, only the reader and his doctors should decide what tests and treatments are relevant and useful in his specific case. The author and publisher specifically disclaim any liability for any loss or risk that is incurred as a consequence of the use and application of any of the contents of this book.

Although the cases presented in this book are true, the names of the individuals have been changed to protect their privacy.

The author has made every effort to provide accurate information such as e-mail addresses, telephone numbers, medical practitioners' offices, and websites at the time of publication. However, the author and publisher do not assume responsibility for errors or for changes that occur after the book is published. Nor do the author or publisher have any control or responsibility over third-party information or the content of websites.

TABLE OF CONTENTS

DEDICATION

To my mother, Dolores Cohen-Levy, who always supported me through every undertaking. When I was 19 and questioning my choice of medicine versus becoming a writer, she said, "Why can't you do both?" I didn't think it was possible, but time proved her right.

INTRODUCTION

A BETTER APPROACH
TO PROSTATE CANCER

"It's hard to know what to do when you don't know what you have."

I learned I had prostate cancer on December 6, 2011. My urologist, a highly experienced and knowledgeable doctor, recommended surgery or radiation therapy for my disease. As a writer, I am always open to a new idea for a book, but I decided against writing about my prostate cancer. I didn't want to think about it any more than necessary. I wanted to get treated and move on with my life.

And so, two weeks later I met with Dr. Frederick, the prostate surgeon. As he described the details of prostate removal surgery, or prostatectomy, in which he would remove the entire prostate gland, he asked me: "Do you want me to take out one or both neurovascular bundles?"

The neurovascular bundles contain the nerve and artery trunks to the prostate gland. Cutting them could render me impotent or incontinent, possibly both, perhaps for the rest of my life. I was too dumbfounded to answer.

The doctor continued, "Your cancer is on the left side, so we should definitely take that bundle out. If we don't, there's a 30% greater chance of your cancer returning. Still, to give you the best chance of getting all of it, we should take the right bundle too." He paused for a second then asked, "What do you want to do?"

Dr. Frederick was intelligent, experienced, calm and personable. He had performed more than five hundred robotic prostatectomies, the treatment most often recommended for prostate cancer. Based on his demeanor and attention to detail, I figured he was a good surgeon.

What did I want to do? My left brain struggled for an answer while my right brain recoiled and cringed. I had been diagnosed with prostate cancer two weeks earlier, and everything I'd heard since then sounded worse and worse.

Dr. Frederick assured me that over time most men get some return of normal sexual and urinary functioning, but what did "over time" and "some return" mean? Although I was a doctor, I wasn't a urologist or oncologist (cancer specialist), and I was as overwhelmed as any of the other 240,000 American men who face this situation each year.

THE PRESSING URGE TO JUST GET IT OVER WITH

Listening to the doctor speak so calmly about mutilating my body seemed unreal. This was serious, permanent, no turning back stuff. I imagined being single at 66, impotent and incontinent. I couldn't fathom it. On the other hand, I imagined dying slowly, agonizingly of prostate cancer. Tough choices.

I weighed the odds Dr. Frederick had given me. Part of me wanted to halt the debate in my head and simply say, "Okay, let's get it over with!" I figured I probably wouldn't become both impotent and incontinent. I'll be okay, I told myself. Empty words. I was in deep denial. I could not perceive myself as other than what I had always been. I'd had surgeries before and came out fine.

Suddenly I heard myself saying, "Let's do it."

Surely I had PTSD, posttraumatic stress disorder. It doesn't take a war to cause PTSD. Mine began with the C word, and now with Dr. Frederick's graphic prostate removing, nerve severing descriptions, my PTSD was peaking. I am not the only one to react this way. Heart attacks and suicides double after men receive a diagnosis of prostate cancer.[1] You can see why.

Fate rescued me from my urge to rush ahead. The hospital's prostate surgery schedule was backed up three months. They would call me. I told them to move me up if there was a cancellation. I wanted to get it over with because until then I would just worry about how much cancer I had, whether it had already spread, whether I made the right choice, whether I would be impotent or incontinent or both for the rest of my life, whether the surgery would save my life or ruin it, and so on, around and around in my mind.

A LACK OF DETAILS

The next day, when I could think again, my mind was beset with questions. The main one: How could I make an informed decision about surgery and whether to sever the neurovascular bundles with so little information? Was there any other area of medicine that demanded such dire decisions with so little data? Here's one example: surgery was not recommended for men whose cancer had already spread beyond the gland. With my cancer score low (more on this in Step 2), spread wasn't likely, but we didn't know for sure. If I underwent surgery and metastases were found, then the surgery would be for naught, and I might be left impotent and incontinent anyway.

The whole process seemed so backward, so 20th century. With good reason, I realized, because it is the same method we've used since 1990. Before then, prostate cancer assessment was even more primitive.

At this point I knew the following: my PSA level was high at 15 ng/ml (nanograms per milliliter), then on repeat 13.4. A normal PSA is 4 ng/ml or less. These high PSA levels meant surgery or radiation was necessary. My biopsy showed a low-grade cancer on the left side of my prostate gland. However, because biopsies frequently miss areas of cancer, the cancer could also be on the right side, and it may have already spread, too. We didn't really know.

On digital rectal exam, my prostate was smooth without any tumors palpable along the posterior side of the gland. This was good, yet the cancer could have spread in a different direction beyond the reach of the doctor's finger. The cancer could be huge on the forward, anterior side of the gland, and we would not know it.

Multiple prostate surgeons told me that these questions do not matter because if the biopsy detects one area of cancer, other cancers likely exist elsewhere in the gland. Pathology examinations of men's prostate glands after surgical removal proved this. Therefore, the only reliable treatment was the complete removal of the prostate gland by prostatectomy.

This is what many urological surgeons say to their patients. In other words, the way the system works is that the doctors doing the biopsy and delivering the diagnosis are almost always urologists, many of whom are prostate surgeons. Hence, most men receive the recommendation one would expect from a prostate surgeon:

prostatectomy. Yet more and more today, experts disagree with this approach. Not every diagnosis of prostate cancer requires aggressive treatment. As *Prostate Cancer 2014* will explain, other and often safer options do exist for the great majority of men diagnosed with prostate cancer.

If you have been recently diagnosed with prostate cancer, you may be thinking like I did, go ahead, cut out the damn cancer and be done with it. Yet even if you agree to surgery or radiation therapy, these are not always cures. The cure rate for these methods is around 75%. The cancer returns about 25% of the time.

The other disturbing fact is that in doctors' efforts to eradicate all degrees of prostate cancer, prostate surgery or radiation is frequently recommended and performed on men who don't need these aggressive treatments. It is estimated that *of the nearly 100,000 American men who undergo radical treatment for prostate cancer each year, 85,000 do not actually need it.*

Where did I stand in this continuum? At this point, I didn't know. My work in medicine has included general medicine, pain research, psychiatry, psychopharmacology, and research into how to prevent the side effects that kill 150,000 and hospitalize 1,000,000 Americans a year. What did I know about prostate cancer? Very little.

I asked my urologist, "Can we do other tests to better clarify the picture? Perhaps an MRI?" This standard test is performed in the diagnostic workups of people who undergo surgery on their knees, lungs, hearts, brains, and just about everywhere else in the body. Why not the prostate?

"Unfortunately, MRIs are not helpful for prostate cancer," Dr. Summers, my urologist, explained. "The prostate is situated so deep in the pelvis, the MRI is not able to give us a clear picture of prostate cancer."

NEW TESTS AND NEW POSSIBILITIES

Three weeks later, I was having lunch with a group of men, none of them doctors, but instead prostate cancer survivors. I learned from them that advanced diagnostic tests do indeed exist, and the fellows encouraged me to get them. These men had been where I was now, with a cancer diagnosis and a frightening lack of details.

I got the tests, and the results changed everything for me. Six weeks from the day I received my diagnosis of cancer, I finally knew what I had, where it was, and whether it had spread. I also learned that with my low grade cancer, I had time to deliberate about the best way to proceed. In fact, most men diagnosed with prostate cancer have time to obtain other tests and other opinions and to consider multiple treatment options. In the great majority of men, prostate cancer is slow growing and slow to spread. There usually is time to obtain a thorough medical assessment, which most men with prostate cancer do not receive today. And there is time to consider other, less invasive treatments that can remove a localized cancer with far less damage, which most men today never hear about.

Unfortunately, when men receive the diagnosis "cancer," their instinct is to decide quickly and try to get rid of it as soon as possible. Family members tend to think the same way. This is why so many men choose aggressive therapies such as prostatectomy or radiation treatment, each of which can cause serious, often life long damage to a man's sexual functioning or bladder control.

THE STANDARD DIAGNOSTIC APPROACH FOR PROSTATE CANCER TODAY

The problem with this approach is that it provides inadequate information and leads to the overtreatment of 85,000 men annually. This is how it usually goes:

1. Elevated PSA levels and/or abnormal digital rectal exam will lead to...
2. A "blind" biopsy. If positive, you have cancer. If negative, another biopsy may be recommended...
3. A diagnosis of cancer will lead to...
4. A recommendation for prostatectomy or radiation therapy.

Sometimes, men are given a third option, watchful waiting. Watchful waiting means waiting passively, which is unacceptable to most men. Men diagnosed with cancer want to do something. That's how I felt and why I placed myself on the surgery schedule. I did not want to spend the rest of my life watching and waiting and worrying about the cancer within me.

The root of the problem is that PSA levels and biopsy specimens are just not sufficient for making an accurate diagnosis of a man's prostate cancer. Yet these are the only tools that doctors have had for the last twenty-four years and that they continue to rely on today for recommending treatment options to 240,000 men a year. When you understand the inadequacy of PSA levels and biopsy results for making accurate diagnoses, coupled with doctors' determination to not let any man die from prostate cancer, it becomes clear why so much overtreatment occurs with this disease.

A BETTER APPROACH

The day of all or nothing—radical treatment or no treatment—is ending. A better approach exists, and it is already being used in many of the most highly respected medical centers in the United States. Steps 1 through 6 of *Prostate Cancer 2014* take you through the new diagnostic process I recommend, with the tests you need to obtain and where you can get them. Step 7 describes genetically-based tests that are available now for improving the accuracy of prostate cancer biopsy interpretations, for determining the aggressiveness of a man's prostate cancer, and for identifying the most effective drugs for high-risk prostate cancer. The introduction of genetic tests represents another breakthrough, a quantum leap in diagnosing and treating prostate cancer, and many more genetic tests will be coming soon. Step 8 describes the C-11 PET/CT scan, a huge advancement in the early and accurate detection of metastatic prostate cancer.

If you follow the steps I outline, you will acquire a full picture of your disease: where it is, how large it is, and whether it has spread. These are essential questions that must be answered yet most prostate cancer evaluations today do not answer them or even try to. This may be because many urologists are not aware of, or not convinced about, the new tests I describe, so your doctor may not mention them to you. Many of you will have to learn about these new methods on your own, from a support group, from other doctors, from web surfing, or from this book.

Most doctors are sincere, yet many are conservative and cautious about change. In researching my books and medical articles on medication side effects and how to prevent them, I learned long ago that new ideas take far too long to be accepted and implemented in the health care world. It can take ten to twenty years for a new idea or method to be verified by studies, accepted by medical leaders, approved by their governing associations, and reimbursed by insurance companies. If you rely only on what your doctor tells you, you may not learn about and obtain the new tests you need to fully know what you have. Like me, you will be asked to make an all or nothing decision about treatment with insufficient information.

Once you know the nature and extent of your prostate cancer, making a decision about treatment becomes much easier. Section 2 discusses the broad range of 12 treatment options now available for men with prostate cancer. These options include aggressive therapies such as prostatectomy (Option 1) and four types of radiation therapies (Options 2-5), as well as newer focal therapies such as cryotherapy (Option 6), focal laser ablation (Option 7), and HIFU (high intensity focused ultrasound, Option 8).

Options 9-12 comprise the non-invasive therapies including medication treatment (Option 9) and active surveillance (Option 10), which is a process of observation coupled with regular, frequent testing for men with low grade cancer. Option 11 discusses alpharadin, a non invasive treatment for men with metastatic bone disease. Option 12 describes finasteride (Proscar), a drug that obtained recent attention as a preventive for prostate cancer, but as I explain, there is a big downside.

Section 3 contains two chapters. Step 9 (What Does Your Data Say?) explains how to organize your test results and make a decision about treatment. Step 10 offers 30 questions you can ask your doctor. The questions are listed in categories, some appropriate at your first visit, others for when you are making choices about diagnostic tests, and the remainder about treatment options. The questions are merely suggestions. You may not need to ask every one of them, and there may be other questions you want to ask about the specifics of your individual case.

A 21ST CENTURY APPROACH TO PROSTATE CANCER COMING SOON

Prostate cancer is the most common cancer (other than skin cancer) in men. It can be a deadly disease, killing 30,000 men in the U.S. and 280,000 men worldwide each year. Because of this, every case of prostate cancer today is treated as deadly. Yet, approximately 85% of men with prostate cancer will not die of it, so treating every case as deadly has led to massive overtreatment and much unnecessary, often permanent pain. In the past, we have treated every case as deadly because we have lacked a way of separating the dangerous cancers from the non-threatening ones. This is why performing surgery or radiation on so many men with prostate cancer has been the accepted course of treatment. Until now.

With the new tests available today, this one-size-fits-all method is no longer necessary. As prostate cancer oncologist Dr. Mark Scholz says:

"Only about one out of seven men with the disease—perhaps 15%—are truly at risk. New research shows that there is an indolent variety of the disease that is not life threatening, a type that can be safely monitored without immediate treatment. The tragedy is that most men don't know this." [2]

How can you find out if you are in this 85% group that does not require depressive intervention? This is what *Prostate Cancer Breakthroughs 2014* explains.

The problem with the current medical method is that it hasn't caught up with the new advancements. To make the right decision, you need to have the right information. For men with prostate cancer, no easy treatment options exist. All have risks. This is why it is so important for you to obtain all of the tests necessary for defining your cancer, and as many second opinions as you need to know all of your choices.

Medically and legally you have a right to complete knowledge of your situation. This right is called informed consent, a right written into the medical code. I have written about this issue many times. The fact is that patients rarely obtain adequate informed consent, and this is certainly the case today for most men with prostate cancer. This is why I finally decided to write *Prostate Cancer Breakthroughs*, to pass along what I learned and to tell you about the new tests and treatments you can get today.

With the emergence of these new diagnostic tests and treatments, a renaissance in prostate cancer care is quietly underway. It is a large wave, building slowly now, that will hit the shore in full force later in this decade. Just as the last decade saw great progress in the medical approach to breast cancer, major breakthroughs are now on the verge of irrevocably changing our approach to prostate cancer.

The problem for you, as it was for me, is that if you have been diagnosed with prostate cancer, you can't wait for the renaissance in prostate cancer care to fully unfold. You can't wait for your doctor to get up to speed in a year or two or five. You have prostate cancer now and must make decisions now.

I encourage you to take the time now to learn about these breakthrough options in prostate cancer diagnosis and treatment. The information can expand your choices and change the course of your care for the better, as it did mine.

SECTION 1

THE KEY: A MORE ACCURATE DIAGNOSTIC APPROACH

STEP 1

WHY YOU MUST GET
AN ANNUAL PSA TEST

Nearly thirty thousand men die each year from prostate cancer. This number will climb to roughly 55,000 over the next few years. Why? Because in 2013, government panels and medical associations decided to no longer encourage PSA testing for any man, not even men with a higher risk for developing the disease. Hard to believe, isn't it?

How did this happen? In early 2012, the United States Preventive Services Task Force recommended that doctors should abandon routine PSA testing in healthy men.[1] Their reasoning: elevated PSA (prostate specific antigen) levels lead to too much unnecessary treatment that causes serious, permanent harm. The task force was referring to the tens of thousands of unnecessary prostate biopsies, surgeries, and radiation therapies that doctors rush men toward based on elevated PSA levels. The USPSTF was correct about the rampant overtreatment of men with prostate cancer, but rejecting PSA testing was like ordering doctors to put their heads in the sand, as if the disease would simply disappear.

In 2013, other prestigious organizations jumped on the anti-PSA bandwagon. This included the American Urological Association, which in May 2013 released its in-depth report on PSA testing. The AUA told doctors to discontinue routine PSA testing for all men 40 and older. For men at higher risk, such as men with blood relatives with histories of prostate cancer as well as African-American men, the association meekly suggested that they discuss the benefits and risks of PSA testing with their doctors.[2] Of course, with doctors already being told by the AUA to dispense with routine PSA testing, this is probably what most doctors will tell these higher-risk men.

To me, the AUA's approach is not a solution. It is a retreat to the past, to the 1980's, before PSA testing began. It is true that thousands of men are rushed each year to radical, often damaging treatment when elevated PSA levels are found. This is why I wrote *Prostate Cancer Breakthroughs*: to inform men about the newer, better options that can allow them to avoid overtreatment and still obtain proper treatment when it is necessary.

In June 2013, a timely study was published in the *Journal of the American Medical Association* on this issue. The study demonstrated that the overtreatment of men diagnosed with prostate cancer is a serious problem affecting tens of thousands of men—and it is getting worse.[3] Yet, the problem isn't the PSA test itself. The problem is system that is tragically outdated in its approach to diagnosing and treating prostate cancer.

PSA: ITS VITAL ROLE IN THE EARLY DETECTION OF PROSTATE CANCER

Abandoning PSA testing is shortsighted for another reason: it is irreplaceable today. No other test is as simple, convenient, inexpensive and proven for the early detection of prostate cancer.

In the 1980s, before PSA testing commenced, the main method of diagnosis was from a digital rectal examination of the prostate. By the time the cancer could be felt, it was well advanced and frequently untreatable—and 50,000 men died annually from prostate cancer. In the 1990s, with PSA testing, 30,000 died annually. PSA testing saved 20,000 men each year from slow, painful deaths from prostate cancer.[2] PSA testing produced a breakthrough in the early detection of prostate cancer. And they are telling us to stop doing this test?

This is why many experts have spoken out against the new guidelines and in favor of continuing annual PSA testing. These experts warn that if routine PSA testing is abandoned, deaths from prostate cancer will rise significantly back to pre PSA levels, which amounts to an additional 25,000 men's deaths a year from prostate cancer. I share this concern.

PSA TESTING IS PROVEN TO SAVE LIVES

PSA is shorthand for prostate specific antigen, a protein released by prostate cells into the bloodstream. It's normal to have a small amount of PSA in your blood, up to 4 nanograms per millimeter (ng/ml). Prostate cancer cells release more PSA than normal cells, so an elevated PSA level can be (but not always is) an early indication of prostate cancer

A study published in the *New England Journal of Medicine* in March 2012 demonstrated unequivocally that PSA testing saves lives. This large study showed that the death rate from prostate cancer was reduced 29% in a study group that received annual PSA testing in comparison to another group that did not.[4] This study confirmed another study published a year earlier with similar results.[5]

These studies provided another astounding statistic: for every 1,000 men who receive PSA testing, one prostate cancer death is prevented. Somehow, the anti-PSA faction interprets this as a reason to stop annual PSA testing. Again, hard to believe.

The PSA test is inexpensive. One thousand men getting a PSA test equals about $22,000. I wish we could prevent a death from breast or colon or lung cancer so inexpensively. The cost of treating a man with terminal prostate cancer is many times more expensive. And first and foremost, beyond the numbers, what is the value of saving a man's life? Of saving 25,000 men's lives annually—the ones that could be prevented but won't be if we discontinue PSA testing.

As we see so often with large bureaucracies, the debate has boiled down to a numbers game. This is not a good way to make decisions that will affect the lives of tens of thousands of men. If the PSA test can save the lives of thousands of American men each year, how can we stop using it? Especially since the problem isn't the PSA test, but doctors who misinterpret an elevated PSA result.

Just last week I was on a National Public Radio show. A man called in and explained that his doctor had recommended radiation treatment for him. "Why did your doctor recommend radiation," I asked. The man explained that his PSA level had increased from 1.7 to 2.5 ng/ml. Understand, these levels are normal, not even close to being abnormal. Although there was no medical basis to do so, the doctor performed a biopsy to look for cancer. The biopsy was normal. And although a more recent PSA level had dropped down to 1.9, nevertheless the doctor advised radiation treatment. I strongly advised the man to get a second opinion.

This case is an extreme example of doctors recommending biopsies and aggressive treatments with no sound medical basis. The regrettable thing is that it happens every day, many times every day. Although urologists are seen as the experts on prostate issues, they treat many other conditions and are trained surgeons. Many are not experts on interpreting PSA results, and many recommend prostate biopsies when they aren't needed.

The PSA test wasn't the problem for the radio caller. His doctor was the problem. Discontinuing PSA testing doesn't solve this problem. Besides, it isn't always the doctors' fault. The PSA test is useful as a general indicator of a prostate problem, but often it is not accurate enough for making treatment decisions. Everyone involved in treating prostate cancer knows that we need a test superior to the PSA, but until it arrives the PSA is far better than nothing.

Meanwhile, research centers across the land are working on a PSA successor. For example, the University of Michigan Health System is now offering a urine test called the Mi-Prostate Score (MiPS). Already validated on 2,000 samples, the PSA test and MiPS together were significantly more accurate than PSA alone for predicting prostate cancer. In addition, MiPS also predicted the level of aggressiveness of the cancer. The test measures not only PSA, but also two genes, TMPRSS2:ERG and PCA3, that are specific for prostate cancer. MiPS is not 100% accurate but may be a significant step forward from PSA alone. UCLA is also developing an improved PSA test called A-PSA. In addition to PSA itself, which indicates prostate cancer cell activity, the test measures six antibodies the body creates to fight prostate cancer (www.urology.UCLA.edu/body.cfm?id=458). A-PSA is still undergoing study and not available clinically.

I am not recommending MiPS or any other advanced test now undergoing study to replace the PSA test. These new tests require the test of time, are expensive, and may not be covered by insurance. However, MiPS is available to the public, so you might want to check it out (www.mlabs.umich.edu).

MOVING FORWARD INSTEAD OF
MOVING BACKWARD

It is said that generals always prepare for the last war, not the next one. And so it seems with the doctors and medical organizations mulling over PSA testing today. The problem is, they have based their decision to dump the PSA test on statistics and treatment models from yesterday. These models we have been using for twenty-four years are the reasons why so many men are sent unnecessarily for aggressive, injurious treatments they don't need. With the new methods I describe in Steps 5 and 6, the decision to halt routine PSA testing becomes short-sighted.

In coming years, men with repeatedly elevated PSA levels will be sent first for advanced diagnostic testing, not biopsies. For the first time, we will have—indeed, we already have!—tests that can sort out the men who need biopsies from those who don't. And the ones who need aggressive treatment from those who don't. These advances will greatly improve our accuracy when interpreting PSA results. This is why I encourage men to obtain PSA testing, because it can save your life!

John's doctor had stopped ordering annual PSA tests. But as part of John's pre-operative evaluation prior to a colonoscopy, the proctologist ordered a PSA. The result was 9, triple John's previous test 3 years earlier. John obtained the tests I talk about in this book and also a biopsy. The result showed prostate cancer that needed immediate treatment. The treatment should extend his years and maybe cure him. Without the PSA test, John would have been like the men before 1990, before PSA testing, whose cancer was often untreatable by the time it was discovered.

So if you are over 50 or over 40 if you are African-American or have a family history of prostate cancer, my advice is to request a PSA test among your blood tests for your annual physical exam. Most doctors will do so if you ask. If you don't get an annual exam, ask your doctor to order a yearly PSA test. Obtaining PSA testing is important not only as a check for prostate cancer, but also to serve as a baseline for comparison with future PSA tests. And keep your own log of your PSA test results.

AN ELEVATED PSA DOES NOT ALWAYS MEAN CANCER

Because prostate cancer cells produce more PSA than healthy cells, doctors get worried when a man has a PSA result above 4 ng/ml. Yet an elevated PSA level does not automatically mean prostate cancer. There are other factors that may cause your PSA to rise. And just because your PSA level is higher than 4 does not automatically mean you must rush to a prostate biopsy.

George, a member of my support group (Step 4), always tells men to think of an elevated PSA level as similar to an engine light signal on your car's dashboard. When it lights up, it indicates a problem but not specifically. Likewise, when your PSA level is elevated, it signals a problem but not necessarily cancer.

One common reason for an elevated PSA is the benign prostate hypertrophy (BPH), which means prostate enlargement, that commonly occurs as men age. The average prostate size of a man age 45 is around 40cc (cubic centimeters). A general rule of thumb is that the PSA level should not exceed 10% of the prostate size, or 4 ng/ml or less in a man with a 40cc prostate gland. As the prostate size increases in some men as they age, their PSA levels may rise too.

Some doctors do not know this and will recommend a biopsy if your PSA level is higher than 4. However, they need to gather more information first. Prostate biopsies can have serious complications (bleeding, infection), another reason one should be performed only if needed. A friend of mine was hospitalized because of a dangerous blood infection from a prostate biopsy. He almost died.

Using my own case as an example, my PSA level in 1996, when I was 51 years old, was 7.1. Most urologists would have immediately recommended a biopsy, but my cautious urologist understood that the high PSA could simply reflect my large prostate. He also knew I had previous prostate infections, which also can elevate PSA levels. The next year my PSA level was 3.7, within the normal range.

My urologist back then ordered another test, the PCA-3, which measures a type of RNA (ribonucleic acid) that is released from prostate cancer cells but not from normal cells. This test can sometimes be helpful in determining whether an elevated PSA represents cancer. Often, however, the results are equivocal and therefore the PCA-3 is not widely used. My PCA-3 result was unhelpful. I watched my PSA levels gyrate up and down for many more years, but until 2011 a biopsy was not necessary.

Other factors that can elevate PSA levels are orgasm within 48 hours prior to a PSA test. So can riding a bicycle or exercise bike, a prostate exam or massage, or other activity that places pressure on the prostate gland, forcing more PSA material into the bloodstream.

If your prostate examination suggests you may have a prostate infection, it should be treated first, and a few weeks after treatment you should have another PSA level drawn. If the antibiotic eradicated the infection, the PSA level may drop back into the normal range. One man's PSA level jumped from normal one year to 37 the next. His doctor thought he had an infection, prescribed antibiotics for 3 weeks, and the level returned to normal. The lesson is: don't panic if your PSA level is suddenly high.

It is important to understand that a single PSA test is not absolutely reliable. Levels of the prostate specific antigen the test measures can fluctuate. You can obtain a PSA test and then repeat it 2 weeks later, and the result may differ. The PSA test's accuracy as an indicator of prostate cancer is considered to be around 75%, not 100%. For this reason, interpreting PSA levels is not always cut and dried. Nevertheless, you should consider any rise in your PSA level significant until proven otherwise, and you should discuss with your doctor whether any of the other causes of an elevated PSA may apply to you.

CAUSES OF AN ELEVATED PSA TEST

- Enlarged prostate (benign prostate hypertrophy)
- Prostate infection
- Orgasm within 48 hours prior to PSA testing
- Pressure on the prostate gland (such as bicycle riding, exercise bike, prostate massage)
- Prostate cancer
- Laboratory error

A major part of the problem of overtreatment is the current method of reliance on PSA levels and biopsy results to make treatment decisions. Until now, doctors haven't had much choice. But PSA and biopsy results are not accurate enough and do not provide enough specific information for doctors to make accurate treatment decisions. We know this now, but the old system continues to prevail: of the 50,000 men who have prostatectomies each year for prostate cancer, over 40,000 are unnecessary. The numbers are similar for radiation therapy.

ALWAYS REPEAT AN ABNORMAL PSA TEST

Some men are biopsied based on a single, slightly elevated PSA test. If the biopsy does not reveal cancer, the urologist may do further biopsies just to be sure cancer hasn't been missed. One expert tells of a man who was biopsied five times based on a single elevated PSA test. The biopsies never found cancer. Turns out, his prostate was huge, 164 cc, as compared with to the average prostate size of 40 cc. The man's large prostate explained his markedly elevated PSA. A repeat PSA test in this man may have shown a lower PSA level.[6]

In July 2009, my PSA was 8.4, the highest ever. Yet my PSA had been bouncing up and down between 1.6 and 7.2 for fifteen years. Was this just another upward bounce or a sign of something more serious? I was worried. My urologist and I agreed to delay a biopsy until we repeated the PSA test. The next result was 4.5, low for me compared to my other PSA results over recent years. We decided to postpone a biopsy.

Time slipped away, and I did not check the PSA until two years later—poor judgment on my part! My PSA was 15.3, nearly double my previous high. I knew this was serious. Not even my large prostate could explain a result this high. I had another PSA test, and it came back high too: 13.4. My prostate size was 75 cc, which inflated the result somewhat, but even when I corrected for this, my PSA levels were still high and nearly double the levels from 2009. This was a red flag I could not ignore. A doubling of PSA numbers within two years is a worrisome sign. That's when my urologist used the B word: biopsy.

THE IMPORTANCE OF A DIGITAL RECTAL EXAM

By the time you are reading this book, you probably have had a digital rectal exam (DRE). If not, and your PSA level is high, a DRE should be done. The doctor will insert a gloved finger into your rectum and feel your prostate. Before he does so, make sure he spreads plenty of lubricant on your anus. Then tell him to give you a few seconds warning, take some deep breaths and exhale slowly, thereby relaxing your muscles as the doctor inserts his finger. Keep taking slow deep breaths to keep your muscles relaxed until the DRE is over. DRE only takes about 20 seconds.

Why is the DRE important? First, the doctor can feel the surface of the posterior aspect of your prostate gland, feeling for any irregularities, bumps or elevations. Eighty-five percent of prostate cancers occur in the posterior area. A prostate with a smooth posterior wall is a good sign. Irregularities are important because they may indicate cancer.

With a DRE, your doctor can get a sense of the overall size of your prostate. If your PSA is elevated, it is important to get more precise information. Before starting the DRE, ask your doctor to also perform an ultrasound test (known as a TRUS for transrectal ultrasound) that will accurately measure the size of your prostate. Most urologists have this device.

It is estimated that 50% of prostate biopsies in the U.S. are performed because of elevated PSA levels in men with benign prostatic hypertrophy (enlargement).[6] This is why it is important to know your actual prostate size. If it is large enough to explain your elevated PSA level, you may not need a biopsy.

My DRE was normal in December 2012, but my PSA numbers had been consistently high. Even if I factored in the other possible causes of my elevated PSAs, they were not enough to explain PSAs of 15 and 13. There was no escaping the fact I needed a biopsy.

STEP 2

BLIND BIOPSY, TARGETED BIOPSY OR NO BIOPSY?

Why is a prostate biopsy necessary? A biopsy is the only way to directly examine prostate tissue and to determine whether cancer is present. Thus, a prostate biopsy is essential for men whose PSA levels or digital rectal examination suggest the possibility of prostate cancer.

If cancer is found, the pathologist will study the tissue, identify the type of prostate cancer, and grade the level of aggressiveness. No other test can provide this information. This is why the biopsy is such an important procedure in the diagnosis of prostate cancer.

SHOOTING IN THE DARK: THE BLIND BIOPSY

In my case, I went ahead with the biopsy because it was clear from my PSA numbers that one was needed. In retrospect, I should have waited for further testing, but at the time I did not know there were other tests that could guide the biopsy needle to the most suspicious areas of my prostate. Equally important, I was anxious to learn if I had cancer. You may feel the same way. Most men do.

Dr. Summers did a good job. A prostate biopsy is unpleasant but mine was not as painful as I expected. Dr. Summers numbed the area and took fourteen samples from various areas of my prostate, following a deliberate pattern. The one problem with my biopsy was that it was blind.

"Amazingly, prostate cancer is being diagnosed today almost exactly the way it was twenty-five years ago. Prostate biopsy is being performed in a systematic but blind manner." Daniel Margolis M.D., Department of Radiology, UCLA.

By "systematic," Dr. Margolis means that today's standard biopsy is performed following a grid pattern that was developed a couple of decades ago. This is the best most doctors can do because they have no tests indicating where the cancer might actually be. So when Dr. Summers performed my biopsy, he was shooting in the dark. This is why blind biopsies miss about 20% of prostate cancers. Many of these men will then have to undergo a second or third blind biopsy, because their doctors want to be as sure as possible that they have not missed prostate cancer. With our current methods, there is no way for doctors to know for certain whether prostate cancer is present or not. That's why this type of biopsy is called "blind."

Some doctors are so concerned about missing prostate cancer, they perform a procedure known as a saturation biopsy in which they take 20 or 30 prostate samples while the man is under anesthesia.

THE DOWNSIDE OF A PROSTATE BIOPSY

For urologists, a prostate biopsy is a standard procedure, part of their daily practice. It is no big deal. Dr. Summers did warn me about the possibility of excess bleeding or infection, but I was not warned that these adverse effects could be severe enough to require the hospitalization, mostly for blood infection, in 2 to 4% of men after biopsy. One in a thousand men die.[1,2]

Another significant risk of prostate biopsies is currently under-appreciated. With 1.2 million prostate biopsies done annually in the U.S., tens of thousands of low-risk cancers are discovered.[3] In fact, by age 50, 30% of men have cancer cells in their prostate. By age 80, 50% have prostate cancer cells. These cancers are usually low-risk and will not harm the great majority of the men. Yet many of these men receive aggressive treatment anyway. In the United States, a diagnosis of prostate cancer leads to aggressive treatment 80% of the time, even in men who are diagnosed with low-risk cancer, the type that experts agree can be followed without invasive treatment. This method of observation is known as active surveillance (Step 10).

All of this confusion and overtreatment are the result of one problem: our inability to reliably differentiate dangerous prostate cancers from non-threatening ones. Until now, if your blind biopsy revealed cancer, doctors have had to assume you had a life-threatening cancer unless proven otherwise. This is why so many men are treated aggressively (often over-aggressively) with prostatectomy or radiation therapy. The great fear of urologists is to assume a cancer was non-threatening, only to have it spread and kill a man. PSA levels and biopsy results are simply not adequate for making accurate treatment recommendations for thousands of men. With few tools to tell the doctor otherwise, all cancers had to be considered high-risk. If I were an urologist, I might feel the same.

If you have any question about whether a biopsy is necessary, do not hesitate to get a second opinion, preferably from an urologist in an unaffiliated office or health system or a prostate oncologist (cancer specialist).

THE TARGETED BIOPSY

The traditional method of performing prostate biopsies is already beginning to change. Now in selected medical centers, for the first time we have tests that allow us to see inside the prostate gland. These new tests, especially the DCE (dynamic, contrast enhanced) MRI, can locate areas of possible prostate cancer within the gland itself. If done before your biopsy, the tests can inform your doctor where to direct the biopsy needles. The advantages of this new type of targeted biopsy is that fewer needles are needed, trauma to the prostate gland is reduced, and accuracy of results is improved. As doctors begin to learn about this method, the targeted biopsy will become the standard of care. This will make today's blind biopsies and saturation biopsies under anesthesia things of the past.

However, this new method is not yet available everywhere, nor has it been integrated into the methods of most urologists today. Don't be surprised if your doctor has not even heard about the targeted biopsy.

Today, targeted biopsies are being performed at many of the cancer centers using the new, DCE-MRI. These centers are listed in Step 5. Doctors who perform color Doppler ultrasound testing can use this in-office method to perform targeted biopsies. These doctors are listed in Step 6. Please note that the color Doppler ultrasound is different than the standard ultrasound device that most urologists have for measuring the prostate gland.

Progress continues in the development of better methods for doing targeted biopsies of the prostate gland. In 2013, UCLA introduced a method for combining MRI and advanced Doppler ultrasound technology to produce a three dimensional "fusion" image that is now being used for performing targeted biopsies.[4] An excellent 6-minute video explaining the method can be viewed at the UCLA website: http://urology.ucla.edu/body.cfm?id=455. This MRI-Fusion technique is also being used at the LIJ-North Shore Medical System in New York: http://www.northshorelij.com/hospitals/news/image-guided-fusion-biopsy-prostate.

OR NO BIOPSY?

One morning in September 2013 I was speaking with Robert, a 67 year-old former surgical assistant at a major hospital and now an artist. "I have been following my PSA levels for many years," he told me. "It used to be 1.75 but gradually rose to 3.5. Last March, it jumped to 8.4. The doctor said I needed a biopsy. I was shook up. From my former work, I'd learned that one shouldn't rush into surgical interventions. I found your book. It really enlightened me. I have had two severe prostate infections in previous years and suspect I still have some inflammation down there. I took some anti-inflammatory supplements and told my doctor I wanted to repeat the PSA test before we made any decisions. A month later, the PSA was 3.4."

"With your previous prostate infections," I told him, "you should be cautious about letting a doctor biopsy your prostate unless there are no other alternatives. You are high-risk for a prostate infection after a biopsy. Taking antibiotics before and after the biopsy may protect you, but may not. Four percent of men develop infections severe enough to require hospitalization after prostate biopsies, and nearly one in 1,000 die."

I recommended the advanced diagnostic tests I discuss in Steps 5 and 6. These would determine whether a biopsy was necessary. "If your PSA jumps up again, do the tests first, before anyone sticks a biopsy needle in you. The tests can tell whether there is anything worth biopsying."

One of my patients in my psychiatry and psychopharmacology practice, which I do one-third time (I research and write the other two-thirds), saw *Prostate Cancer Breakthroughs* at Amazon.com. He asked me about his father, age 76, who had undergone repeated annual biopsies of his prostate gland. "They diagnosed him with prostate cancer several years ago but told him it is low-grade and will probably never harm him. As part of the surveillance, his doctors require a prostate biopsy once a year. My father dreads them. He says they are very painful. He would do anything to avoid a biopsy."

Most experts now agree that prostate biopsies are performed far too often. Does this mean that prostate biopsies should never be done? Prostate biopsies are essential for accurately identifying and grading prostate cancer. My criticism of our current method of biopsing men suspected of having prostate cancer is not about the biopsy itself, but that approximately half of the 1.2 million prostate biopsies performed annually in the U.S. are unnecessary.

I have come to believe that whenever a doctor recommends a prostate biopsy for a man, other tests, especially the new, prostate DCE-MRI (Step 5), should be performed first, if possible. These tests can tell the doctor and the man whether there are any suspicious areas in the prostate worthy of a biopsy. If the tests reveal suspicious areas in the prostate gland, then the biopsy can be targeted toward these areas instead of being done blindly. A targeted biopsy is much more likely to retrieve adequate amounts of suspicious tissue and to answer key questions about diagnosis. A targeted biopsy may also require fewer biopsy cores overall, thereby reducing the pain of the procedure, the trauma to the prostate gland, and the risk of post-biopsy bleeding, infection or other adverse effects. And if the advanced prostate DCE-MRI shows no suspicious areas, then the biopsy may be withheld.

Samir Taneja M.D., of the NYU Langone Medical Center, states, "The prostate remains the only organ in the body that doctors will biopsy without good imaging. In every other organ, biopsies are directed by imaging to a specific location." The doctor added that at his medical center, "We now routinely do MR imaging on every newly diagnosed prostate cancer patient to help us in both assessing risk and directing treatment." You can see Dr. Taneja's video at http://prostate-cancer.med.nyu.edu/test-diagnosis/biopsy-and-diagnosis.

MRI-guided biopsies are being implemented at several top medical centers in the U.S. (Step 5). And for men like my patient's father who require an annual biopsy to monitor prostate cancer, the new tests may also reduce the necessity for many of these biopsies. After all, if the DCE-MRI does not show any change in the man's cancer or any new areas of suspicion, and if the PSA tests have remained level, a repeat biopsy may not be needed.

Yet, just to be clear, if you need a prostate biopsy because of high PSA levels or other reasons, and you cannot get a guided biopsy, then get the random one that is more commonly available today. One man spent a year trying to learn about the targeted biopsy. Meanwhile, his PSA level went from 6 to 9 to 11. Even when I encouraged him to obtain a biopsy as soon as possible, he wanted to put it off a few more months so he could take a long vacation. Apparently he did not realize the worrisome significance of his rising PSA levels. Maybe he was in denial. The moral is: if you need a biopsy, get it. A targeted biopsy is preferable if you can obtain it, but if not, get a blind one.

TABLE 2.1: YOU MAY NEED A PROSTATE BIOPSY IF …

1. An abnormality is felt on digital rectal examination, or
2. Your PSA level is repeatedly high, or
3. Your PSA level is 4.0 or less, but the level has doubled in one year or less, or
4. Your abnormal PSA levels cannot be adequately explained by an enlarged prostate, prostate infection, or other factors, or
5. The new tests, DCE-MRI (or Parametric MRI) or Color Doppler Ultrasound, identify areas in your prostate suggestive of cancer. These tests allow for a targeted biopsy, a safer and more accurate method than today's standard blind biopsy

---

PROSTATE CANCER GRADING

Of the fourteen biopsy specimens that Dr. Summers took from my prostate, four showed cancer, all on the right side of the gland. The pathology report summarized my cancer stage as "T1c."

The "T1" meant that the cancer was found within the prostate via a surgical intervention. The T1 grade also implies that the doctor was not able to feel the cancer on digital rectal exam (DRE). The subtypes of the T1 grade are:

- T1a = The cancer was found unexpectedly during a pathology examination of tissue removed from surgery for an enlarged prostate.
- T1b = Found unexpectedly as above, the cancer involves more than 5% of the removed tissue.
- T1c: Cancer found on biopsy.

The next higher grade, T2, means that the cancer was found during a DRE.

- T2a: On DRE, cancer involves less than 50% of one lobe of the prostate.
- T2b: On DRE, cancer in more than 50% of one lobe of the prostate.
- T2c: On DRE, cancer exists in both lobes of the prostate.

When the DRE indicates that the cancer has spread outside of the prostate gland, the stage is T3.

- T3a: On DRE, cancer has spread outside of the prostate on one side.
- T3b: On DRE, cancer has spread outside of the prostate on both sides.
- T3c: On DRE, cancer has spread into one or both seminal vesicles, two pouches that hold semen located just above the prostate gland.

The T4 stage means that on DRE, the cancer was found to have invaded other nearby structures.

- T4a: On DRE, cancer found in the bladder, urinary sphincter, or rectum.
- T4b: On DRE, cancer has spread to other structures such as lymph nodes, pelvic wall or muscles.

THE IMPORTANCE OF THE GLEASON SCORE

The Gleason Scoring System is used to describe the appearance of the prostate cancer cells when viewed under a microscope. Low-risk cancers look similar in many ways to normal prostate cells, whereas high-risk cancer cells have lost the normal organization of prostate cells and appear aggressive.

The Gleason score is determined by examining prostate tissue retrieved from biopsy. The pathologist evaluates the size, shape, and appearance of the normal prostate cells and cancer cells, and then classifies the type of cancer and its level of abnormality. Prostate cancer cells with a mild degree of abnormality are given a Gleason score of 3. Cancer cells with a high degree of abnormality receive a score of 5.

The total Gleason score represents the sum of two grades. The first is the grade given to the most prominent pattern of cancer cells in your biopsy specimens. The second grade is given to the second most common pattern of cancer cells. Sometimes the pathologist sees only one cancer pattern, but sometimes more than one pattern is present.

Most men whose biopsies show prostate cancer receive Gleason scores of 6 to 10, representing less aggressive to more aggressive degrees of cancer, respectively. A Gleason score of 6 indicates a consistent pattern of low-grade cancer, scoring a grade of 3 on both Gleason assessments. Gleason 6 is the most common score for newly discovered cases of prostate cancer.

Another common Gleason score is 7. This score is a bit more complicated in that it sometimes indicates a 4 for the most common pattern of cancer cells and a 3 for the next most common pattern. However, a Gleason 7 can also indicate a 3 + 4 pattern. The distinction is important. A 3+4 means the most common cancer pattern is 3, the lowest grade, whereas a 4+3 means the most common pattern is 4, an intermediate grade cancer. These distinctions can be important when making treatment decisions with your doctor.

My Gleason score of 6 indicated that my cancer had a low level of risk. Still, cancer was clearly identified. A Gleason 6 score is less worrisome than the higher scores, yet it is still cancer and can kill. Dr. Summers, my urologist, urged me to consider surgery or radiation as soon as possible. Thinking these were my only alternatives, a week later I met with Dr. Frederick, the prostate surgeon. (I described our meeting in the Introduction.)

TABLE 2.2: THE MEANING OF GLEASON SCORES

Gleason grades can range from 1 to 5 for each side of the prostate gland; then the top two scores are added together for the final Gleason score (2-10).

Gleason 1:   Cancer cells look almost normal.

Gleason 2:   Cancer cells appear almost normal but early cancerous changes are apparent.

Gleason 3:   Some cells are clearly cancerous to a mild degree and have some degree of irregularity.

Gleason 4:   Many cells display cancerous abnormalities and are crowding out normal cells.

Gleason 5:   No normal prostate cells remain, and cancer cells are highly abnormal.

THE ULTRASOUND

As soon as Dr. Summers finished taking the biopsy samples, he inserted a small ultrasound device and measured my prostate size. The proper name for this procedure is a Trans-Rectal Ultrasound or TRUS. My prostate measured at 75 cc, almost twice the average 40 cc size for men my age. The ultrasound test was needed, but it should have been done two weeks earlier when Dr. Summers performed the digital rectal exam. When trying to interpret my high PSA levels, it would have been helpful to know that I had a 75cc prostate gland.

Even now, Dr. Summers did not explain how the size of my prostate affected the interpretation of my PSA numbers. It was my new support group friends who explained this and a lot more to me, changing the course of my care.

STEP 3

ASSESSING YOUR FINDINGS

You have now finished the standard diagnostic tests for prostate cancer: PSA levels, digital rectal exam, and biopsy. If you are following the standard model, you will be asked to make a decision about treatment. In the standard model, your choices are all or nothing: prostatectomy or radiation therapy, which destroy the entire prostate gland, or watchful waiting, which amounts to doing practically nothing. If you have advanced prostate cancer, your choices may differ, such as radiation therapy plus hormone suppression therapy or chemotherapy. As you can see, there are no happy choices in the old model.

Yet whatever your situation, you may have more diagnostic and treatment options that you have been told. The first step involves assessing the diagnostic information you already have. The first question is: based on the Gleason score, *what grade of cancer do I have?* If, like me, your Gleason score is 6, you may fit into the low or intermediate-risk group.

Then the key question is; *which risk category?* The survival statistics between the two groups differ significantly, and so do the treatment options. For example, if you are in the low-risk category, active surveillance may be a safe choice and also allows you to avoid surgery or radiation. If you are in the intermediate risk group, surgery or radiation or other invasive treatments become more likely options.

PSA FINDINGS

If your PSA results are between 4 and 10 ng/ml, you may fit into the low-risk group. My case was atypical in that my two PSA results were 15.3 and 13.4 ng/ml. These numbers were significantly elevated, well over the 10 ng/ml ceiling for the low-risk category. I was in the intermediate risk category, defined as PSA levels between 10 to 20. Even if I factored in my large prostate, I was still in the intermediate-risk group, just slightly above the low-risk ceiling. If your PSA levels are above 20, you may be in the high-risk group.

DIGITAL RECTAL EXAM FINDINGS

A normal digital rectal exam is required for inclusion in the low-risk group. Inclusion in the intermediate-risk group requires a normal DRE or a single, palpable small nodule. Multiple nodules or one large nodule would place you in the high-risk group.

NUMBER OF BIOPSY CORES POSITIVE FOR CANCER

Another important factor in risk assessment is how many cancerous cores were obtained from your biopsy. Usually twelve cores are taken, and inclusion in the low-risk group requires zero to two cores (0-17%) positive for cancer. Sometimes fewer or more than twelve cores are taken. My urologist took 14 cores, and four were positive (29%). Yet one core contained just 1% cancer, hardly worth counting, I decided. Three cores out of fourteen (21%)—did this equal two cores out of twelve? Not quite. Again, I was in the intermediate-risk category, which requires 3-6 cores out of 12 to have cancer, but at the low end of the category. If more than 50% of your cores have cancer, this would place you in the high-risk category.

GLEASON SCORE

This score rates the degree of abnormality and apparent aggressiveness of the cancer cells. A Gleason 6 or less is required for inclusion in the low-risk group, Gleason 7 for the intermediate-risk category, and Gleason 8 or above for high-risk.

Because the Gleason scoring of the cancer in your biopsy cores is so crucial, some experts recommend always getting a second opinion. Gleason scoring is a subjective process that depends entirely on the eye and experience of the pathologist. Studies have shown that variations can occur in Gleason scoring from one pathologist to another, even when they evaluate the same specimens.

TABLE 3.1: WHAT IS THE RISK LEVEL
OF YOUR PROSTATE CANCER?

Low-risk
- PSA less than 10 ng/ml
- Less than 3 biopsy cores (out of 12) with cancer
- 0 biopsy cores with more than 50% cancer
- Clinical stage of T1 or T2a
- Gleason score 6 or less
- Digital rectal exam normal.

Intermediate-risk
- PSA 10-20 ng/ml
- 3-6 (out of 12) biopsy cores with cancer
- Clinical stage T2b or Gleason score 7
- DRE normal or small nodule.

High-risk
- PSA above 20 ng/ml
- More than 50% of biopsy cores with cancer
- Clinical stage T2c or Gleason score above 7
- DRE reveals large or multiple nodules.

HEADING FOR TREATMENT?

Hopefully, your findings place you into one of the well-defined groups, so that you can determine your next step. Even then it is not always that simple. Or perhaps you have findings that fit different risk groups. My PSA and biopsy cores said intermediate-risk, but my Gleason score and normal DRE said low-risk. This raised questions for me but not for Dr. Frederick, the surgeon. "Two high PSA levels, 4 cores—this places you squarely in the intermediate-risk category," he said. "You are not low-risk or a candidate for active surveillance. You need surgery. "

I heard him. After all, Dr. Frederick had done more than 500 prostatectomies. He had vast experience in removing prostate glands and then, after the gland was dissected by pathologists, seeing how much cancer they actually contained. In many cases, far more cancer is discovered in prostate glands when dissected following a prostatectomy than initially indicated by the biopsy. This is why urologists lean toward aggressiveness in recommending surgery. They want to be sure to get all of the cancer right away.

I understood Dr. Frederick's point of view. The only findings that argued otherwise were my normal DRE, which didn't mean much once the biopsy found cancer, and the Gleason 6 score. The Gleason 6 was the most important single finding of all, because it indicated that my cancer was early and slow growing. This alone, however, could not guarantee my safety.

Trying to clarify my picture further, Dr. Summers, my urologist, ordered bone and CAT scans. These tests can be helpful in high-risk cases, for they can determine whether the prostate cancer has spread to bone, lymph glands or other tissues near the prostate. They are used most often with men who have PSA levels above 20 or Gleason scores indicating aggressive cancers. (These scans are now being superseded by a new, more accurate test, the Carbon-11 PET/CT scan, approved by the FDA, in 2013—see Step 7).

My scans were negative, fortunately, but this did not change my risk status. I was at intermediate risk, although in my opinion not by much. At this point, I had pretty much decided on treatment. The only question was: prostatectomy or some form of radiation therapy?

Just then, new, hopeful ideas emerged from an unexpected source. No matter whether you are low, intermediate or high-risk, you must check out this source before making any final decisions.

STEP 4

THE VOICE OF EXPERIENCE: THE SUPPORT GROUP

As mentioned earlier, in their haste to rid themselves of prostate cancer, many men rush right into treatment. You may be tempted to do so, but consider this: Neither surgery nor radiation is a guarantee of cure, and with either treatment you run the risk of serious, permanent side effects. Besides, because prostate cancer is very slow growing in most cases, you have time to do some research on your own.

Many men do not realize that they don't have a full picture of their disease. Many accept at face value what their urologist tells them and never consider obtaining a second opinion. Many urologists are good doctors, but they are surgeons and are trained to look at things from a surgical perspective. With this disease, second opinions can be helpful and sometimes quite enlightening.

Unfortunately, most men do not bother going to a support group. Why? Most men do not think they need support. For some men the idea of seeking support implies emotional weakness. This is what I thought after being diagnosed. Yet I went anyway and learned that a good support group can offer far more than support. It can provide important information you will not get anywhere else.

MY LITTLE UNOFFICIAL SUPPORT GROUP

Two weeks after meeting with the surgeon, I sat down for lunch with seven prostate cancer veterans. Over several meetings, this small support group played a pivotal role in increasing my knowledge of my disease, which in turn decisively altered my decision about treatment. Without this group, I would have had a prostatectomy in January 2012. From the questions they raised and the tests they told me about, I realized there was far more diagnostic work to be done and far more treatment options to consider.

Fortune played a role in my meeting this group. Dr. Summers, the urologist, sent me to a nurse specialist who did a good job of providing information about the standard treatment options, answering my questions, and then suggesting the hospital's prostate cancer support group. Because it was December and the group was not meeting that month, she also told me of a nearby independent support group, the Informed Prostate Cancer Support Group (IPCSG). I had pretty much decided on prostatectomy, and I had spoken to two men who had done well with the surgery, so I thought I had enough information. Why should I bother finding out what other men had to say?

Still, knowing that the more information I had about prostate cancer, the better, I called IPCSG and left a message. The next day, I received a call from a leader of the organization. IPCSG was not meeting in December either. Indeed, I have never been to a regular meeting, because they meet on Saturdays, when I work. However, there was a small group of men who met informally for lunch once a week. Although all of the men were members of IPCSG, their small group was not formally affiliated with the organization. I had lunch with them the following week.

Many prostate cancer support groups serve as a meeting place where men can share information and tips about how to handle the long-term impacts from surgery or radiation therapy. These groups serve a useful purpose. However, my little group functions differently. Most of the three to ten men who show up for lunch each week, as well as others who drop in occasionally, are past the recovery stage. Some have had prostatectomies, others radiation. One has had both. Some are on chemotherapy. Some are in apparent remission. Others continue to struggle with problems of impotence or incontinence, others with recurrence of their cancer, and others are coping with side effects from their testosterone suppressing or anti-cancer drugs.

The meetings consist of the men updating each other on their status, latest test results, or treatments they are considering or already receiving. The men also spend time discussing new information in news reports, online or in the medical literature. These are educated and assertive men, who before retiring held important and demanding jobs. For their work, they had to know their stuff, and they now know their stuff about prostate cancer. They spend considerable time reading current studies, contacting institutions and experts around the country, and obtaining details about new therapies that go beyond what we find in typical public relations press releases.

The fellows in the group were the first to explain how my large prostate and my earlier prostate infections could contribute to my high PSA levels, information my urologist never mentioned. They were the ones who pointed out that the huge jump from my PSA level of 13.4 in December to 22 in January, which worried me greatly, was probably from the biopsy four weeks earlier, another fact my urologist neglected to explain. And they answered my questions about what more could be done to better define the size and location of my prostate cancer, and determine if it had already spread.

These men told me about the latest diagnostic methods such as the advanced prostate DCE-MRI and color Doppler ultrasound, tests that can identify and define prostate cancer within the gland itself. My doctor never mentioned these essential tests, because most urologists do not know about them or there are no nearby facilities that offer them.

I also was able to purchase a dozen DVDs from IPCSG, showing nationally respected experts speaking to the Saturday group on a variety of topics (you can do the same at ipcsg.org.). The DVDs added additional high quality information to my growing fund of knowledge. A good DVD for you to start with is Richard Lam, M.D., speaking in May 2013. If you want to see my talk, it was June 2013, but the one-hour talk doesn't offer nearly as much information as this book contains. IPCSG offers more than 30 DVDs with lectures and Q&As with national experts on a range of topics relevant to our disease.

Most of all, Gene and my other support group buddies helped me put things in perspective. They reminded me again and again that I had time to check things out. I was Gleason 6, wasn't I? Most prostate cancer grows slowly, especially G6, so there was time for me to learn more about my disease and the various treatment options. There was time for me to be thorough, so when I made my treatment decision, there would be no "If only I had…."

PASSING IT FORWARD

Every month or so, newly diagnosed men appear at our lunch meeting. Like me, these men are worried and confused about how to make vital decisions regarding their prostate cancer. We answer their questions and impart information as best we can. None of us are experts, so our goal is not to direct their cases or make decisions for them, but to merely let them know their options for diagnosis and treatment, something they rarely obtain in full elsewhere.

Every man's case is different. You may not be interested in joining an ongoing support group, but I think it is helpful to take the opportunity at least once to speak with men who have previously walked the path you are now walking. Most men get a lot of support from family and friends, and useful information from their doctors, but there is nothing like speaking with men who have been through it.

Different support groups offer different formats. You may find that you prefer a formal, moderated group that provides speakers, allowing you to do more listening than interacting. Or you may feel more at ease with a group of men in a casual environment. No matter the kind of group you choose, a group can offer practical advice and tips, resources to help you better manage your situation, and feedback about the doctors the men have seen or heard speak.

Some men join us for lunch one time and do not return. That's okay, because there are no expectations or obligations. We keep meeting because we enjoy it, we like helping newly diagnosed men and each other, we're always coming across new science to discuss, and because we all have a chronic condition known as prostate cancer that can change and evolve over time—and all that aside, we like and respect each other. The fields of prostate cancer diagnosis, testing and treatment are evolving so fast now that our group never suffers from a lack of issues to talk about. And with so many men keeping an eye on developments, we can keep up with things as well as, or sometimes better than, many of the doctors.

That said, I hope you decide to try a prostate cancer support group. Whether you go once or several times, learn as much as you can from the men. Add their input to the information you have received from your doctors, your reading and other sources. When it is time for you to make a treatment decision, your thoroughness will serve you well.

Another resource is Gene, IPCSG's contact person and Chief Operating Officer, who has volunteered to respond to your calls and answer your questions. You can reach him at 619-890-8447 or gene@ipcsg.org. Gene is not a doctor and cannot provide medical advice. Gene is a 12-year survivor of prostate cancer and has had a lot of experience communicating with men newly diagnosed or experiencing recurrence. He can provide helpful information on many of the issues that concern men diagnosed with prostate cancer.

STEP 5

THE DYNAMIC, CONTRAST-ENHANCED, PROSTATE MRI (DCE-MRI)

Y ou are probably familiar with the test known as the MRI (magnetic resonance imaging). Although MRIs have long been used as vital diagnostic tests for orthopedic, gastrointestinal, pulmonary, brain and other conditions, MRI technology has not been useful for identifying cancer in the prostate gland. Because the gland sits so deeply in the pelvis, and because with PSA testing prostate cancers are initially very small, MRIs have been unable to obtain a clear enough picture to differentiate prostate cancer from normal prostate tissue.

"I think imaging is really the future in cancer care in every organ," says Samir Taneja M.D. "Up until recently, imaging did not allow us to see prostate cancer. These cancers are microscopic, so seeing them on an x-ray or film of any sort is almost impossible. One of the reasons the surgeons remove the whole prostate gland is because we haven't known where the cancer really is. If we can now treat patients through image guidance, then our treatments could be far less radical in some patients than they are now."

MRI technology employs strong magnetic fields and radio frequency impulses translated by computer into highly detailed pictures of internal body structures. The MRI was one of the great advances in medicine in the late 20th century, and the technology keeps evolving and improving today. Some experts, including me, believe MRI technology has advanced to the point of use for prostate cancer. Dr. Summers, my urologist, had no faith in this test and was unwilling to write a prescription for me to get one, even if I went outside my health care system and paid for it myself.

The majority of urologists today probably agree with Dr. Summers. Gerald Chodak M.D., author of *Winning the Battle against Prostate*

Cancer, has excellent credentials and is very knowledgeable. In his 2011 book he states, "At present, there is not enough proof that the MRI should be done routinely [for prostate cancer] but research is ongoing to find out."[1]

THE MEDICAL SYSTEM IS SLOW TO ACCEPT NEW TECHNOLOGY

Dr. Chodak may be right about one element. It is true that we lack published studies convincing enough to persuade today's doctors to order DCE-MRIs (or parametric MRIs) for prostate cancer patients. But I was diagnosed with prostate cancer at the end of 2011, and I could not wait for some medical authority or insurance panel to grant approval five or ten years down the road. For decades I have been writing and lecturing about the difficulty people have in obtaining individualized care in our huge medical-pharmaceutical complex. My emphasis has been on prescription drugs. For example, when Prozac was introduced in 1988 at a one-size-fits-all 20 mg starting dosage, it greatly helped some of my patients, yet provoked serious side effects in others. My research uncovered evidence that 5 mg was all that many patients needed. Because the only pill was a 20mg capsule, I had patients dump out half or three-quarters of the contents. Many of them did great on these lower dosages. It took the manufacturer a decade to finally market lower dose pills.[2] In the medical world, sometimes you cannot wait for the system to catch up with what is known and needed now.

The usual complaint from doctors is that they practice evidence-based medicine, and if they do not see enough evidence to convince them, or if their medical association has not yet approved a new test, they will not recommend it. However, in my experience, most doctors do not know what the term evidence-based medicine actually means. In my research and writings about why medications cause more than 100,000 deaths and 1 million hospitalizations in the U.S. each year, I point out that "proof" differs in meaning to doctors and to patients.[3] Many doctors think evidence-based medicine means proof from large, placebo-controlled clinical studies, like the ones done by drug companies. Doctors readily dismiss any other type of information as inadequate or anecdotal, a word they often use with derision.

Yet evidence-based medicine encompasses all types of information including large studies, small studies, individual case reports, and personal experience.[4-8] Doctors often scoff at case reports or personal accounts, yet these are what the FDA uses to identify toxic drugs and ban them. If such reports are good enough for the FDA, they are good enough for me. And if eight intelligent, well-informed prostate cancer survivors in my group tell me about a new MRI that can accurately identify prostate cancer in the gland, I am going to check it out. I might discover they were wrong, or maybe they were right. Either way, it could not hurt to be thorough. At that time I was hovering between a diagnosis of low-risk versus intermediate-risk prostate cancer. Right then, prostatectomy or radiation therapy seemed the likely choices for me, but I would rather avoid both, providing it would not jeopardize my survival. If another test could shed more light on my case, I welcomed it. So should you.

If you think about the factors I discussed in the last chapters—PSA levels, biopsy cores with cancer, Gleason score—none of these provide information on the location, size or extent of a man's prostate cancer. Perhaps an advanced prostate DCE-MRI might help clarify whether a man has low-risk or intermediate-risk cancer—as the test did for me. My thinking going in was, even if the MRI showed cancer throughout my prostate gland, then I would know specifically what I had and undergo surgery or radiation with an accepting mind.

The advanced prostate MRI cost $550 out of pocket. It was a bargain.

THE ADVANCED PROSTATE MRI: A BREAKTHROUGH TECHNOLOGY

The MRI machines I have seen for prostate imaging are newer, wider, and not as deep as the old, coffin-like versions. A contrast material, gadolinium, is injected intravenously before the exam begins. The blood vessels of cancerous prostate tissue absorb gadolinium more readily than normal prostate cells, thereby making the cancerous tissue visible. This type of MRI is known as a Dynamic Contrast-Enhanced MRI. In some centers, a sensor is placed inside the rectum to provide further clarity to the picture (make sure they use plenty of lubricant). This type of MRI is known as an endorectal MRI. Another type is the multiparametric MRI, which provides more data than the others. In my experience, the differences between these tests are slight, and any of them can be very helpful in identifying cancer in the prostate gland. For the remainder of this book, I will refer to the test as the DCE-MRI, although the specific test used by different centers may vary. You will have to be specific about this DCE-MRI with your doctor, because many health systems use the standard MRIs to rule out metastases near the prostate gland, but this older MRI cannot see into the gland itself. Many doctors are not aware of the new DCE-MRIs and will think you mean the latter. A friend of mine went to an Ivy League medical center. He had a high PSA and asked the doctor for a DCE-MRI. The doctor sent him for a standard MRI. The doctor did not know the difference.

The rating of my DCE-MRI machine was 1.5 Tesla. Tesla is the measurement of the magnification quality of a MRI machine's magnetic field. Until recently, 1.5 Tesla was the highest strength available. The new 3.0 Tesla MRI machines, with their greater magnification of microscopic structures, are now being used at many medical centers. However, the resolution of the MRI machine is not the only key factor in identifying prostate cancer. One of my group members received a 3.0 Tesla MRI at the local university, but it could not identify his prostate cancer because it lacked the sophisticated software needed to do so. Several centers now possess advanced prostate MRI 3.0 Tesla machines, and you should choose this if possible. If not available, a 1.5 Tesla MRI will usually do.

I received the results from the radiologist the next day. He wrote:

The test has identified a right sided and posterior peripheral zone tumor larger than 1 cc. in size, but small. No extracapsular [beyond the prostate] extension into the seminal vesicles or pelvic metastases.

I sighed with relief. These were the kind of details about my cancer that I had been seeking: size, location, and signs of spread. The cancer size was not tiny, but small, about the size of the tip of my pinkie. It was in the right lobe of the gland. The left lobe was clean. This matched the biopsy findings, which found cancer in the right but not the left. There was no sign of spread to the edge of the prostate gland, seminal vesicles, lymph nodes, bone or elsewhere.

Finally, I had a complete picture of my cancer. This made a huge difference for me, and it can do so for you and most men with newly diagnosed prostate cancer.

HOW RELIABLE IS THE ADVANCED PROSTATE MRI?

Just as PSA levels and biopsy findings are not entirely reliable, the findings with a DCE-MRI are not 100% reliable either. Experts rate the accuracy at 85 to 90%. This is very good, but the DCE-MRI can miss some cancers, especially small ones, those below 5 millimeters in diameter. These cancers could cause trouble eventually, but with close follow-up and repeated tests, these small cancers should be identifiable before becoming a problem.

More and more, I see proof building in support of the prostate MRI. A study published in 2009 concluded: "DCE MRI can accurately identify intraprostatic [within the prostate] cancer foci. Possible applications are guidance for biopsies, selection of patients for watchful waiting, and focal treatment planning."[9]

Dr. Peter Scardino, chief of urology at Memorial Sloan-Kettering Hospital, which specializes in treating cancer, is known for his great skill in performing prostatectomies in the treatment of prostate cancer. About the DCE-MRI, he writes in his book, "It has proven to be the best means we have today for seeing a cancer in the prostate."[10]

When asked how he uses the DCE-MRI results, Dr. Scardino replied, "If I don't see anything on an MRI, it helps reassure me you probably don't have a large, life threatening cancer." Then he added an important statement: "I don't rely just on the digital rectal exam, the PSA, the biopsy results or the MRI. But if we put all that information together, we can get a pretty good idea of what's going on."[11]

Exactly! As it is in many areas of medical endeavor, the basic method is to obtain all tests that can help define the problem. For you and other men with prostate cancer, this means PSA levels, DRE, biopsy, and a DCE-MRI. For me, this MRI confirmed I was low-risk, not intermediate, and suddenly I could consider newer, less aggressive treatment possibilities.

If I had any lingering doubts about the validity of the DCE-MRI, I was convinced when I looked at the following list of the medical centers now using it in their diagnostic evaluations of men with prostate cancer.

TABLE 5.1: MEDICAL CENTERS USING THE ADVANCED, NEW PROSTATE DCE-MRI FOR PROSTATE CANCER DIAGNOSIS

CA: Desert Medical Imaging, Indian Wells
CA: Rolling Hills Radiology, Ventura
CA: Sharp Hospital and Medical Center, San Diego*
CA: University of California, Los Angeles (UCLA)
CA: University of California, San Diego (UCSD)
CA: University of California, San Francisco (UCSF)
CA: University of Southern California, Los Angeles
CA: Veterans' Hospital, La Jolla
CT: Yale Medical Group, New Haven
IL: University of Chicago Medical Center, Chicago
MA: Massachusetts General Hospital, Boston
MD: Johns Hopkins University, Baltimore
MN: Mayo Clinic, Rochester
NY: Memorial Sloan-Kettering Cancer Center, New York City
NY: NYU Langone Medical Center
NY: Sperling Prostate Center, NYC
OH: University of Cincinnati Medical Center
OH: Cleveland Clinic, Cleveland
PA: Fox Chase Cancer Center/Temple Health, Philadelphia
PA: Jefferson Medical Prostate Diagnostic Center, Philadelphia
TX: MD Anderson Cancer Center, Houston
TX: UT Southwestern Medical Center, Dallas
CANADA: Sunnybrook Health Sciences Center, Toronto

*Has a 1.5 Tesla MRI machine; others have a powerful 3.0 Tesla machine.

By the time you read this, the advanced contrast MRI may be available at other medical centers. Check at the major hospitals and cancer centers in your area and perform an Internet search.

A DCE-MRI OF THE PROSTATE
COULD SAVE YOUR LIFE

In a broad article about prostate cancer, the *Wall Street Journal* included a story about Richard, a 54-year-old man who's PSA had doubled within two years, then jumped even higher.[12] This was a large red flag. Richard's prostate biopsy was normal, and the plan was to wait and repeat the PSA test some months later. At the same time, however, Richard enrolled in a study using the DCE-MRI. His test identified areas suspicious for prostate cancer. These findings led his doctor to perform a second biopsy, a targeted biopsy (many of the medical centers listed above facilitate targeted biopsies). Two of the 21 core samples contained cancer. Because the Gleason score was 6, indicating a less aggressive cancer, and the number of positive cores was low, Richard's doctors recommended watchful waiting.

A few months later, Richard obtained a second DCE-MRI. The test showed more cancer, this time larger than on the original prostate MRI, and the cancer was now present on both sides of the prostate. With a complete picture of his prostate cancer condition, Richard decided to undergo a prostatectomy. Based on his findings, I believe he made the right decision. Just think, without the DCE-MRIs, Richard's cancer would have continued growing until later, when it was finally identified by biopsy.

I read Richard's story six months after I had gone through my prostate cancer odyssey. Like Richard, I received differing medical opinions, test results that did not jive, and a DCE-MRI that finally shed much needed light on my situation. For me and for Richard, the DCE-MRI was a game changer. It could also be a game changer for you.

STEP 6

THE COLOR DOPPLER
ULTRASOUND TEST

If you now have your PSA levels, prostate size, biopsy and prostate MRI results, you are ready to talk about treatment options. Then again, you might consider one more diagnostic test that can confirm or clarify the findings you already have. In fact, if the color Doppler ultrasound test were easier to obtain, I would recommend it earlier in your diagnostic process, because it is the easiest way, right there in your doctor's office, to make your biopsy targeted rather than blind.

In my case, I didn't hear about the breakthrough technology known as color Doppler ultrasound until after my DCE-MRI. I didn't think I really needed a color Doppler ultrasound test, but I was still perplexed by the disparity of my high PSA levels and limited DCE-MRI findings. An elevated PSA of 8 or so would have been consistent with my biopsy and DCE-MRI findings, but my PSA levels of 15 and 13 predicted real trouble. This fact was brought home by another test you can use and that many doctors rely on.

If you go to prostatecalculator.org, you will find the Prostate Calculator, a method that determines the risk of your prostate cancer having already spread beyond the gland. All you have to do is input your age, T stage (e.g., T1c), your two Gleason scores (e.g. 3, 3), and PSA level. I inputted my data using my first PSA result, 15.3 ng/ml. The calculator result: a 49.6% risk that my prostate cancer *had already spread outside the prostate*. I was shocked. Spread can mean dead for some men.

Next, I inputted my second PSA level of 13.4. The result barely budged: 47.7% risk of spread. In other words, there was a nearly 50% chance that my prostate cancer had already spread into the seminal vesicles, lymph nodes or bone!

I adjusted my PSA numbers downward by subtracting the impact of my large prostate. Using a PSA result of 10, I ran the number through the calculator again: 42.2% risk of cancer spread outside the prostate! This sounded bad. I thought I was in the clear after receiving the MRI results. The prostate calculator said I was wrong.

I sent an e-mail to a highly knowledgeable member of IPCSG, the local support group I discussed in Chapter 4. He replied that I should ignore the PSA results. The test is only 75% reliable, he said, pointing out that my PSA results were inconsistent with all of my other test results.

I also contacted my internist, who personally called one of the top prostate surgeons in the area. Because of my fifteen-year history of gyrating PSA levels, the surgeon felt strongly that the calculator was probably exaggerating my risk of spread. Nevertheless, risk still existed, she said, and urged me to have a prostatectomy as soon as possible.

I wasn't really seeking more confusion, but there it was. I hope your case is less complicated than mine, but dealing with prostate cancer is not always simple. This is when I decided to go to Los Angeles to see a doctor with expertise in color Doppler ultrasound. I needed confirmation of what I had and what it meant.

COLOR DOPPLER ULTRASONOGRAPHY

Ultrasound is used in many areas of medicine to produce images of internal organs or tissues by bouncing sound waves off of them. In urology, the standard ultrasound apparatus is inserted into the rectum to measure prostate size. This device is called a trans-rectal ultrasound (TRUS).

It is important to differentiate the TRUS machine from the color Doppler ultrasound (CDUS). The latter is an adaptation of the standard ultrasound device. By using advanced computer analysis of the sound waves it generates, the color Doppler device has much greater resolution than standard ultrasound. The color Doppler device is able to measure blood flow within prostate tissue and to translate these findings into color images on a computer screen. Because prostate cancer areas have greater blood flow than normal prostate areas, the cancerous areas produce intensely colored "hot spots" on the screen.

Color Doppler ultrasound is controversial among urologists, partly because they are not trained in its use. And although the technology has been available for many years, the best practices guidelines for urologists do not advocate for the use of color Doppler ultrasound in the evaluation of men with prostate cancer. My personal experience is that it can be quite helpful. If I had learned about color Doppler ultrasound earlier, I would have gone to a doctor who uses it for targeting a biopsy. The doctor can look at the computer screen and aim the biopsy needles at the targets the computer indicates. With a targeted biopsy, fewer cores are often needed. Fewer cores mean less trauma to the prostate gland and less likelihood of bleeding or blood infection. This capability alone should motivate urologists to consider using the device. The accuracy of biopsies would be increased, adverse effects would be reduced, and the necessity for repeat biopsies would be diminished. In some cases, if the color Doppler ultrasound does not identify any sign of cancer, a biopsy may be postponed.

Dr. Duke Bahn, a pioneer in introducing the color Doppler ultrasound in the U.S., explains, "The role of the Color Doppler Ultrasound is in examining the prostate by blood flow pattern (color) in addition to black and white images. In a Color-Doppler study, we pick up about 15-20% more cancers. The Color Doppler Ultrasound also helps us identify the exact tumor size. The tumor size seen on Color Doppler is usually larger than it is in black and white. So the black and white image underestimates the cancer size. In addition, if we see a suspected lesion in black and white and that suspicious lesion shows increased blood flow, it is most likely cancer. The more flow in the lesion, the higher the Gleason grade in general. Then we perform a targeted biopsy rather than a blind systemic random biopsy. A targeted biopsy has a higher yield with fewer tissue cores taken. By getting tissue from the middle of the action, we can get a more accurate Gleason grading. Also, based on the cancer location we can anticipate where the cancer would have spread out, if at all. We can take a tissue sample from the most probable area of cancer escape. By doing so, we can determine the exact stage of the cancer. Since Color Doppler Ultrasound can identify the cancer clearly by the location, size, and blood flow pattern, it can be objectively monitored over the years, especially if someone is undergoing active surveillance.[1]

The color Doppler ultrasound does have some limits in its ability to identify prostate cancer. Like the prostate MRI, color Doppler ultrasound can miss small prostate cancers less than 5 millimeters in size. On the other hand, color Doppler technology has been studied intensively in Japan for more than a decade. Studies show that color Doppler ultrasound can identify 77 to 95% of prostate cancers. In a 2008 study, the accuracy was determined to be 88%.[1A]

MY COLOR DOPPLER ANALYSIS

Color Doppler testing can also serve to provide clarity to a complicated case. This is what I sought in Los Angeles, which was the nearest place with doctors experienced in performing the color Doppler test.

I left San Diego at 5 AM, hoping to beat the LA traffic for my 8:15 AM appointment. Dr. Mark Scholz met with me at the appointed time. Highly regarded in my prostate cancer community, Dr. Scholz is neither a surgeon nor a radiologist. He is an oncologist, an expert in the treatment of cancer with medications. Most oncologists treat many different types of cancer, but Scholz works only with prostate cancer, so he has vast experience in evaluating and treating the disease.

We talked for quite awhile. Dr. Scholz was not fazed by my PSA levels. "Many men do not fit the typical criteria," he assured me. "Believe me, I see many men with much higher PSA levels than yours. The PSA test be the helpful, but it is not always reliable. A high PSA level itself should not dictate your final treatment decision."

Dr. Scholz noted the MRI results. It is a test he orders frequently, and he explained how useful it is to obtain the MRI and the color Doppler test. If the results are consistent, they are highly reliable.

We proceeded with the color Doppler test. Lying on my side on the examination table, Dr. Scholz placed the ultrasound sensor in my rectum. It was uncomfortable but not painful. He placed the computer screen where both of us could see the color images. He showed me the prostate area and pointed to a spot within it. I could see the cancer in exactly the same spot in my prostate gland as the MRI had depicted. The size and shape of the color Doppler image were also consistent with the MRI findings. More important, like the MRI, the color Doppler analysis did not indicate cancer anywhere else. "No cancer in the left lobe, no cancer in the seminal vesicles," Scholz commented.

After the test, Scholz said: "Despite your high PSAs, you are a candidate for active surveillance. This cancer of yours is located in a rather safe area of the prostate gland. It is not near any major structures and shows no sign of spreading beyond the prostate capsule. It is highly likely that this cancer will never bother you."

Music to my ears.

And yet, as I was driving back to San Diego, I remembered an old saying in medicine: the more doctors you see, the more likely you will find one who will say exactly what you want to hear. I believed Dr. Scholz. He was knowledgeable and current in his thinking, and he seemed better informed than the other doctors I consulted about this newly accredited approach, active surveillance. He had written an award-winning book on the subject. To other doctors, interpretation of my results was simple: PSA 15, 4 biopsy cores with cancer = surgery or radiation. Yet Scholz pointed out that my 4/14 cores were not that impressive. He discounted the core that was 1% cancer. This left me with three positive cores, which fit within his criteria for active surveillance.

Still, I had to consider: did I like him because he said what I wanted to hear? Yes, he certainly did that. But his reasoning made sense. I would strongly consider his recommendations.

COLOR DOPPLER ULTRASOUND REDUCES NEED FOR INVASIVE TESTS

In a letter to the *Wall Street Journal*, a man named Frank related his experience with the color Doppler ultrasound. Frank was 74 years old and had benign prostate hypertrophy since age 56. In 1992 his PSA was 5.5 ng/ml. Because the result was above the normal range of 0-4, his prostate gland was biopsied. No cancer was found. Several years later, Frank's PSA jumped to 9.5. Another biopsy was done. It was negative too. Hoping to avoid further biopsies, he obtained color Doppler testing from Dr. Duke Bahn in Ventura, CA, an hour north of LA. Dr. Bahn has published multiple papers on color Doppler ultrasound testing in men with prostate cancer and is considered a pioneer of the technique.

Frank's color Doppler test was normal. In his letter, Frank mentioned that he was unable to find a urologist in the Denver area who performed the color Doppler test. "Every urologist I talked to starts with a biopsy with a high PSA." However, Frank wrote, if the color Doppler test is normal, there should be no need for a biopsy. From his perspective, the current approach did not make much sense. "It seems the medical profession is still in the dark ages regarding examination techniques for benign prostatic hypertrophy and cancer detection,"

Frank continued. "I get the impression that urologists cry 'biopsy!' too quickly and loudly for any PSA above 4.0, no matter what the age."[2]

One million, two hundred thousand prostate biopsies are performed each year in the U.S. Dr. Scholz says this is 600,000 too many. If a color Doppler ultrasound were performed before each prostate biopsy, sometimes it would show no suspicious areas, and the biopsy could be postponed. These men would be followed closely and their PSA levels and other tests would be repeated frequently. Dr. Scholz told me that sometimes the first sign of a developing cancer appears on the color Doppler ultrasound, even while the PSA level remains stable. As one of my group friends says, prostate cancer is an elusive disease. Nothing about it is absolute.

Meanwhile, as the medical establishment awaits studies to confirm the reliability of the prostate MRI and ignores the value of the color Doppler ultrasound, my color Doppler test confirmed the findings of my MRI. That was exactly what I had hoped it would do. While driving home, I thought about how lucky I was to have learned about these tests before rushing into surgery. I now felt fully prepared to consider the many treatment options available to me. And, thanks to the input of my support group, I had more options to consider than I'd known - and you have them, too.

Just to clarify, the DCE-MRI is a more important test that the color Doppler ultrasound. The major medical centers that are already employing the newer methods rely on the DCE-MRI or the more advanced multiparametric MRI. Yet, if you can obtain it, the color Doppler ultrasound can also be helpful for diagnostic purposes as well as for obtaining a targeted biopsy in the doctor's office.

TABLE 6.1: RESOURCES FOR COLOR DOPPLER ULTRASOUND TESTING

Obtained from Internet in, October 2013. Other doctors may offer this test.

ARIZONA
Frank Tamburri ND
Longevity Medical Health Center
Prostate Second Opinions
Phoenix, Arizona
602-493-2273
4wecare.com

CALIFORNIA
Duke Bahn MD
Prostate Institute of America
Ventura, CA
888-234-0004
pioa.org

Douglas Chinn MD
Chinn Urology
Arcadia, CA
626-574-7111
chinnurology.com

Mark Scholz MD & Richard Lam MD
Prostate Oncology Specialists Inc.
Marina Del Rey, CA
310-827-7707
prostateoncology.com

Osamu Ukimura
Keck School of Medicine
University of Southern California
Los Angeles, CA
800-872-2273

FLORIDA
Michael Dattoli MD
Dattoli Cancer Center
Sarasota, FL 34237
877-328-8654
dattoli.com

MASSACHUSETTS
Stephen Scionti MD
Scionti Boston Prostate Center at
    Mass Bay Urology
Milton, MA 02186
617-696-1826
drscionti.com

MICHIGAN
Fred Lee MD
Rochester Urology
Rochester Hills, MI 48307
248-650-4699

NEW YORK
Robert Bard MD
New York, New York 10022
212-355-7017
cancerscan.com

NYU Langone Medical Center
Smilow Comprehensive Prostate
    Cancer Center
135 East 31st Street, 2nd floor
New York, NY 10016
646-754-2400

PENNSYLVANIA
Jefferson Medical Prostate
    Diagnostic Center
Ethan Halpern MD, Director
Philadelphia, PA
215-955-7544

WASHINGTON
Tahoma Clinic North
Seattle, WA 98103
206-402-4215

STEP 7

GENETIC DIAGNOSTIC TESTS FOR PROSTATE CANCER THAT ARE AVAILABLE NOW

Although we have long know that there is a genetic link to prostate cancer—sons of fathers with prostate cancer have a higher risk of contracting the disease—the clinical use of genetic testing for prostate cancer is just beginning. Yet we already have a handful of genetic tests that may vastly improve our methods of diagnosis and treatment. These tests are just the beginning of a new wave of genetically-based breakthroughs that will change our methods for decades to come.

Within a decade, no prostate biopsies will be done without genetic tests that can identify the presence of prostate cancer even when the visual pathology examination identifies none. No prostatectomy will be done without genetic tests to calculate the tumor's aggressiveness and whether immediate further treatment is warranted. No metastatic prostate cancer will be treated without genetic testing to match the sensitivity of the cancer with scores of potential drug therapies.

This chapter describes tests that are already available plus one that is nearing approval. Many, many more tests are on the way. Clinical trials have demonstrated the usefulness of these new tests, yet their accuracy and reliability will ultimately be proven in the clinical cauldron, that is, via their use with tens of thousands of men with prostate cancer. Clinical experience will also separate the most helpful tests from the also rans.

"It's a little tricky to find out which one applies to you and whether it will be paid for by insurance," says Jan Manarite, who runs the telephone help line for the Prostate Cancer Research Institute (http://prostate-cancer.org), a patient education organization.[1]

The tests are already making a difference. Even though they may not yet be perfect, they can add valuable information when making difficult decisions. A *New York Times* article described the case of Angel Vasquez, who wasn't comfortable with his urologist's recommendation of active surveillance. "I said, 'No, my philosophy is if there is something in my body that is not supposed to be there, I want it to come out.'" His doctor ordered a test that showed the cancer was more aggressive than thought. After his prostatectomy, the pathology examination confirmed the accuracy of the test. "Had I left it alone, it would have really progressed," Vasquez said.[1]

Although the shaking out period will take awhile, I find all of these advances incredibly exciting. They are providing us a keyhole's glimpse of an amazing future to come in the medical treatment of prostate cancer and all disease.

TESTS THAT IMPROVE ACCURACY OF BIOPSY INTERPRETATION

These tests are most helpful for men with high PSA levels yet their prostate biopsies are negative. Approximately 1.2 million prostate biopsies are performed each year in the U.S. Of these, 700,000 are determined on pathology examination to be negative (not containing cancer), and 25% of these determinations are wrong—cancer is found on a second biopsy or via other methods. It is easy to understand why this happens. Each core of prostate tissue taken during a biopsy represents just a tiny fraction of the entire prostate volume. The typical random biopsy takes 12 or 14 cores of prostate tissue, less than 1% of the full gland. This is why today's standard blind biopsy misses prostate cancer so often.

A negative biopsy can cause a lot of uncertainty. Is the biopsy result accurate? Is there really no cancer in the prostate gland? Or did the biopsy simply miss a cancer that actually exists? Can the result be relied upon for making life-and-death treatment decisions? If you have a rising PSA level, a negative biopsy result can cause more concern than relief.

In today's medical approach, a negative biopsy often leads to another biopsy. Hundreds of thousands of men each year would be relieved to avoid these additional prostate biopsies, because they all too often prove unnecessary. So is there a better way to tell whether a second biopsy is truly needed? This is the purpose of the following three genetic tests.

Prostate Core Mitomic Test

The Mitomic test is performed on the tissue obtained from your biopsy. Even if your biopsy result has been reported as negative, the test can identify prostate cancer by finding aberrations and deletions in cells' mitochondrial DNA that are consistent with prostate cancer. In other words, although the cells do not appear cancerous upon visual inspection, the Mitomic test can find molecular markers of cancer.

When the Mitomic test is negative (finds no cancer), it is accurate 91% of the time. If the biopsy and Mitomic test are both negative, a second biopsy may not be necessary. Thus, hundreds of thousands repeat biopsies each year might be avoided.[2]

When the Mitomic test is positive for prostate cancer, the finding is accurate 85%-90% of the time. This would suggest a second biopsy, preferably targeted, in order to obtain a cancer specimen for grading and Gleason scoring by a pathologist.

The parent company of the Mitomic test, Mitomic Technology, is developing similar tests for breast cancer, endometriosis, melanoma, and bladder, cervical, thyroid, ovarian and pancreatic cancers. For further information: Mitomicsinc.com.

The ConfirmMDx Test

ConfirmMDx uses patented technology to identify signs of prostate cancer in prostate tissue obtained on biopsy. Even when the visual examination of the biopsy tissue indicates no cancer, this test can find genetic markers in these normal cells suggesting they were near cancer cells in the prostate gland. The test is 90% reliable in determining that a negative biopsy is truly negative, thereby possibly obviating the need for an additional biopsy. If the ConfirmMDx test is positive for prostate cancer markers, a targeted biopsy may be needed to obtain cancer for grading and Gleason scoring. ConfirmMDx has been tested in studies involving over 4,000 prostate cancer subjects.

The parent company of the ConfirmMDx test, MdxHealth, is also developing genetic-based tests for lung and colon cancer. In addition, it is developing tests that can distinguish between aggressive and non-aggressive cancers, and also tests to predict the medications and treatments that are most effective for an individual's cancer. For further information, go to mdxhealth.com.

The QuadVysion Test

With a specialized immunohistochemistry stain, the QuadVysion test identifies a protein present in prostate cancer cells but not in normal cells. The test can be used to confirm that when biopsy material is read as negative, it is truly negative, or to determine if tiny areas of prostate cancer actually exist in some of the biopsy specimens. The parent company of the QuadVysion test, Bostwick Laboratories, also makes another prostate cancer test, the ProstaVysion test, which I discuss in the next section.

No matter whether any of these biopsy specimen tests are positive or negative for prostate cancer, a DCE-MRI should be done before a second biopsy is considered. The MRI can identify a prostate cancer tumor of 0.5 cm or greater and could facilitate a targeted biopsy with its greater likelihood of obtaining cancer tissue for pathology inspection. If the biopsy, the Mitomic or ConfirmMDx or QuadVysion test, and the DCE-MRI are negative, a second biopsy might not be necessary.

You may ask, if a DCE-MRI is done, are these genetic tests necessary? This is a good question. Because the tests are performed directly on prostate tissue obtained from the biopsy, they can tell us about the state of the prostate tissue on a molecular level. For example, if the pathology examination of biopsy tissue is negative and so is the MRI, yet one of these tests identifies prostate cancer markers, what then? One interpretation might be that prostate cancer exists or is beginning to develop in the prostate gland, but it is too early to be detected on MRI. An active surveillance approach might then the adopted.

GENETIC TESTS FOR ASSESSING AGGRESSIVENESS AND ASSISTING TREATMENT DECISIONS

As mentioned earlier, the degree of a prostate cancer's aggressiveness is a key factor in determining a man's treatment. Currently, the Gleason score indicates a cancer's aggressiveness. This score is determined via visual and microscopic inspection of prostate tissue obtained by biopsy. The new genetic tests can allow the Gleason determination to be confirmed on a molecular basis.

The Prolaris Test

A prognostic test for measuring the aggressiveness of a man's prostate cancer, the Prolaris test measures the frequency of tumor cell division in the prostate cancer tissue obtained from biopsy or prostate surgery. The test measures RNA expression levels of genes related to cellular proliferation. The faster the rate of cell division and proliferation, the more aggressive the prostate cancer, and the higher the Prolaris score.

The Prolaris test does not measure whether you have prostate cancer, but how fast your cancer cells are dividing. The Prolaris website states: "Two patients with the same PSA and Gleason scores may have a very different estimate of mortality risk when their Prolaris score is included in their evaluation."

The Prolaris test is intended to help men with low-risk prostate cancer and their doctors decide whether they are a good candidate for active surveillance or should consider an intervention. The test is also used for men who've had a prostatectomy. In the latter case, the Prolaris score can help determine if further treatment, such as radiation therapy, is needed after the surgery.

If you have low-risk prostate cancer, a low Prolaris score may support your choice of active surveillance. If the Prolaris score is high, you may want to choose a more active approach.

The Prolaris test has been examined in four clinical studies involving hundreds of patients each. In each study, the Prolaris test was shown to be a statistically significant predictor of clinical outcomes in men using active surveillance and in men who had received prostatectomies. Over ten years, the test has demonstrated 97% accuracy. For further information: Prolaris.com.

The OncotypeDX Test

OncotypeDX analyzes the RNA from genes in prostate cancer tissue obtained from biopsy and prostatectomy. This approach reveals a gene signature that can help predict your cancer's level of aggressiveness.

In a study of 395 men with prostate cancer, the OncotypeDX test led to the reclassification of 35 men originally deemed low-risk to an even lower risk category, thereby allowing the men to choose active surveillance with greater certainty. Conversely, in the same study 10% of men defined as low-risk were reclassified into a higher risk category, allowing the men to consider other treatment options.

The OncotypeDX test can also be helpful in determining whether further treatment is necessary after a man has undergone a prostatectomy. If the test indicates a cancer that is more aggressive than indicated by the pathology examination, post-operative radiation or androgen blocking therapy might be considered. For further information: myprostatecancertreatment.org.

The ProstaVysion Test

For determining the aggressiveness of prostate cancer from tissue obtained on biopsy, the test's methodology involves the identification of two major mechanisms of prostate carcinogenesis: gene fusion/translocation and loss of a key tumor suppressor gene. The approach includes a projection of your long-term outcome based on analyses published in the medical literature. For further information: bostwicklaboratories.com.

The Decipher Test

For men after having a prostatectomy, the Decipher test determines the activity of a score of prostate cancer genes to assess the likelihood of the cancer returning and spreading. The results can help high-risk men and their doctors know whether radiation and/or androgen deprivation therapy should be initiated soon after the prostate surgery.

In studies, the Decipher test allowed for the reclassification of 60% of high-risk men into a lower risk category. Based on the test, their risk of metastases was low, so they could wait before deciding on further treatment. In contrast, in another subgroup the risk of developing metastases was markedly elevated, and additional treatment was recommended. In this way, the Decipher Test could prove very helpful for men and their doctors in making accurate treatment decisions following prostatectomy. As of September 2013, the Decipher Test was pending FDA approval. For further information: genomedx.com.

Caris Molecular Intelligence Profile and Profile Plus Tests

Performed on tumor tissue from any source, the MI Profile test identifies thirty cancer biomarkers and determines the likely response to treatment with each of 46 FDA-approved cancer drugs. This method is particularly helpful for difficult to treat prostate cancers such as the uncommon, hard-to-treat small cell prostate cancer, or for the more typical adenocarcinoma cancer that is unusually resistant to standard chemotherapy. The "Plus" test performs an advanced sequencing panel for testing an additional 44 biomarkers for matching more drugs. Moreover, the manufacturer, Caris Life Sciences will attempt to match patients with ongoing clinical studies. For more information: carislifesciences.com.

In broad perspective, the recent development of genetic tests to improve three major areas of prostate cancer diagnosis—biopsy interpretation, cancer aggressiveness grading, and the matching of drug therapies for each man's prostate cancer—is amazing. The big question remains: How accurate are these tests today? There is no doubt that in time we will have accurate tests for each of these categories and more. Will some of today's tests prove highly reliable? Or will they all the replaced by better tests that are being developed right now?

Bottom line, no matter the stage and Gleason category of your prostate cancer, it is certainly worth investigating these tests. Ask your doctor. Go to the websites I have listed above. Do a search on the Internet. Be sure to access the Mayo Clinic website about its new genetic endeavor: the Prostate Cancer Medically Optimized Genome-Enhanced Therapy (PROMOTE) study (http://mayoresearch. mayo.edu/center-for-individualized-medicine/prostate-cancer-study.asp). Its purpose is to analyze the genetic characteristics of each man's prostate tumor and predict the most effective treatments. You can also watch a video on this at http://youtube.com/watch?v=LFaI2xAaj7g.

The Mayo Clinic effort seems similar to the purpose of the Caris Molecular Intelligence Profile test. Will it be better than the Caris test? Time will tell.

The University of California, San Diego, which is my university, has recently established a Center for Personalized Cancer Therapy at its Moores Cancer Center (http://cancer.ucsd.edu/care-centers/personalized-therapy/Pages/default.aspx). "Our goal is to transform cancer therapy by using advanced technological tools to predict who will respond to a specific treatment, and to match each patient with the best drug for a particular tumor." The center will treat patients with many other types of cancer including prostate cancer.

Soon, centers like these will be popping up everywhere. This is very encouraging. The momentum is building and appears unstoppable. My gosh, we are learning to use a cancer's own genetics against it! Soon we will be designing specific, genetically designed molecular missiles against the cancer instead of crude, side-effect prone drugs.

Suddenly, the decades' old unfulfilled promise, *a cure for cancer*, does not seem so beyond comprehension. Of course, cancer is a cagey enemy, or nature will come up with something else. Still, the next decades will be remarkable in transforming the treatment of prostate and other cancers toward the molecular and atomic levels. Ideas like this used to be called science fiction, but now it is only a matter of time until they become real.

STEP 8

THE NEW, CARBON-11 PET/CT SCAN FOR METASTATIC PROSTATE CANCER

In late 2012, the FDA approved the use of a new Carbon-11 choline PET/CT scan. This advanced form of scanning is a major breakthrough in our ability to better identify prostate cancer metastases in men with aggressive cancer (Gleason 8-10). The new scan can allow doctors to determine whether men with aggressive cancer already have metastases before making decisions about initial treatment with surgery or radiation. In men whose prostate cancer has already spread beyond the gland, prostatectomy is contraindicated because removing the prostate will not remove all of the cancer. Treatment will therefore involve radiation to the prostate gland as well as to areas of metastases, or medication therapy, Alpharadin therapy (Option 11), or a combination of therapies.

The key advantage of the new Carbon-11 PET/CT scan is that it can identify prostate cancer metastases earlier and with better accuracy than current techniques. The scan is specific for prostate cancer cells, which it can distinguish in bone, lymph nodes, and seminal vesicles, a small structure just above the prostate gland.

With the new scan, much smaller metastases can be recognized, thereby making diagnosis sooner and treatment more capable of cure. Unlike other scans, the Carbon 11 scan identifies heightened fat metabolism, a sign that reflects the heightened metabolic activity of prostate cancer cells in comparison to normal prostate cells. Current methods for identifying metastatic prostate cancer include ultrasound, biopsy, CT scan, standard MRI, bone scans, but none of these is as able to identify prostate cancer recurrences as the Carbon-11 PET/CT scan. The other tests show changes in bone that may represent metastatic prostate cancer, but may also be from other causes. The Carbon-11 PET/CT scan uses a radioactive isotope that lights up only when it binds with prostate cancer cells. Hence its ability to locate metastatic disease earlier and with greater accuracy.

CARBON-11 PET/CT SCAN FOR PRIMARY PROSTATE CANCER

Research on this scan has mainly been directed toward men with signs of cancer recurrence after surgery or radiation treatment. The Carbon-11 Choline PET/CT scan that the FDA approved is being used at the Mayo Clinic in Minnesota for this purpose.[1] However, the use of a similar method, the Carbon-11 Acetate PET/CT scan, is also being studied for initial diagnosis of aggressive cancers by Dr. Fabio Almeida at the Arizona Molecular Imaging Center in Phoenix. I wrote to Dr. Almeida asking about this application for primary evaluation. He replied:

> In addition to running the protocol with C11-Acetate for detecting recurrence, we have been running a protocol to answer the question you have asked. We are using C11-Acetate in those who are about to undergo surgery who have higher risk features on their biopsy: Gleason grade of 7 to 10, a PSA greater than 10, or a large amount of prostate cancer in the gland. The goal is to determine if C11-Acetate PET can help detect prostate cancer metastases in lymph nodes or bone that would alter the treatment plan. We are seeing good results, but the study is in its very early stages.

Dr. Almeida enclosed a 2013 article published in the Journal of Nuclear Medicine. The study concluded, "In patients planning for or completing prostatectomy, carbon-acetate PET/CT detects lymph node metastases not identified by conventional imaging and independently predicts treatment-failure free survival." [2]

A LONG-AWAITED ADVANCEMENT IN DETECTING METASTATIC PROSTATE CANCER

After a man receives treatment for prostate cancer, his PSA level should drop considerably because all of the prostate cancer cells have been removed by surgery or killed by radiation. For example, after prostatectomy, the PSA should drop below 0.2 ng/ml and remain below this level. After radiation therapy, the PSA should drop below only 2 ng/ml. After these procedures as well as after HIFU, cryosurgery, laser therapy or other treatments, a rising PSA may indicate a recurrence of the cancer.

Recurrence of prostate cancer after treatment is not rare. Recurrence rates after prostatectomy are about 25% after ten years. Recurrence rates are slightly higher following radiation therapy.

When the PSA rises repeatedly, it is imperative to identify the location of the recurrent prostate cancer. Did some of the cancer cells survive in the gland when it was bombarded by radiation? Or in the remaining prostate bed after prostatectomy? Or is the recurrence from prostate cancer cells that have spread to local lymph nodes, to the seminal vesicles or bone or other distant areas?

CASE REPORTS ON THE UTILITY OF THE CARBON-11 PET/CT SCAN

Dr. Almeida provided these case reports in the December 2012 Newsletter of the Patient Advocates for Advanced Cancer Treatments Organization (PAACTUSA.org), an excellent resource for men with prostate cancer.

When a man's PSA level began to rise 9 years after prostatectomy, his doctors directed radiation to the area of the prostate bed. Nevertheless, his PSA kept rising. A Carbon-11 Acetate PET/CT scan identified a lymph node with cancer in the left pelvis. No other cancerous lesions were seen. This time, radiation was aimed at the correct area, and the man's PSA dropped to 0.9. This substantial drop in PSA indicated that the Carbon-11 scan had accurately identified the metastatic cancer and that the radiation treatment had been successful.

After radiation, a man's PSA level dropped to 0.43 ng/ml, but 4 years later his PSA climbed again to 3.9. A Carbon-11 Acetate scan identified a suspicious area on the right side of his prostate gland. With this information, a targeted biopsy revealed the cancer, and brachytherapy (pellet radiation) was performed. The man's PSA level decreased to 0.6.

Twelve years after brachytherapy and external beam radiation (forerunner of IMRT), a man's PSA level had risen from 0.16 to 2.17 ng/ml. Carbon-11 Acetate scan identified a single, suspicious lymph node in his upper pelvic area. Surgical intervention removed 13 lymph nodes, and the node identified by the scan was found to have metastatic cancer while the other nodes did not. In other words, the identification of this node by the scan was accurate. After removal, the man's PSA level dropped to 0.19.

Nine years after prostatectomy, a man's PSA rose to 4.8. Carbon-11 Acetate scan identified a single metastasis in a bone in the cervical (neck) spinal area. No other metastases were identified in bone, lymph node, or prostate bed areas. Radiation was directed at the lesion, and the PSA dropped to 0.2 ng/ml.[1]

No other testing or scanning method today could have identified these lesions this early and accurately.

THE AVAILABILITY OF THE CARBON-11 PET/CT SCAN

Because Carbon-11 scans require an on-site cyclotron, this technique is available at only a few centers in America:

> Carbon-11 Acetate PET/CT scan, Arizona Molecular Imaging Center, Phoenix, AZ, Dr. Fabio Almeida, director. http://clinicaltrials.gov/ct2/show/record/NCT01304485, or call 602-331-1771.

> Carbon-11 Acetate PET/CT scan, University of Kansas Medical Center: www.rad.kumc.edu/nucmed/Research/c11.htm.

> Carbon-11 Choline PET/CT scan, Mayo Clinic, Rochester, MN. Director Dr. Edwin Kwon. http://www.mayoclinic.org/choline-c-11-pet-scan/about.html.

This diagnostic method is most effective in men when the PSA level is high or has been climbing. False positive tests, which indicate cancer inaccurately, can occur.

SECTION 2

A Broader Range of Treatment Options For Men With Prostate Cancer

There is an old saying in medicine: The more treatments there are for a disorder, the less likely any of them work well. Put another way, if one treatment for prostate cancer were highly effective with little downside, no one would choose the others. Today, no prostate cancer therapy is anywhere near 100% effective, and each comes with a substantial downside.

Fortunately, prostate cancer is usually a slowly developing disease. Most men have time to gather opinions from doctors, obtain the necessary tests, and speak with men who have been through this difficult process. Gather your information about the various treatments as thoroughly as you can. Consider all appropriate options. Sometimes it may seem like TMI (too much information!), but when you look back at this time in your life, you don't want to regret not having been thorough enough.

Even if you have high-risk disease, it still is worthwhile to obtain all relevant the tests and be painstaking with your doctors in analyzing the results. Even with high-risk prostate cancer, different doctors have different ways of proceeding. It pays to learn all that you can and to get second opinions to obtain new perspectives.

The following eleven options provide information about the treatments used today for prostate cancer, the first ten of which I considered one by one. These chapters are just a start. Dozens of books and hundreds of medical journal articles have been written on prostatectomy and radiation therapy, and new chapters are now being written on emerging new therapies such as proton beam radiation, cryotherapy, laser ablation and so on.. If any of these interest you, you can find plenty of information on the internet, including published medical papers and descriptions provided at websites of doctors and medical institutions providing these therapies. All of these sources of information should also be accessed by men interested in testosterone inhibiting drug therapy or prostate cancer chemotherapy.

A. AGGRESSIVE THERAPIES

OPTION 1

PROSTATECTOMY

Today, prostate surgery plays the leading role in the treatment of men diagnosed with prostate cancer. More than fifty thousand prostatectomies are performed in the United States each year. Most of these are radical prostatectomics, surgeries that remove not only the prostate gland but also the seminal vesicles and, when necessary, adjacent nerve bundles. Most prostatectomies today are done with robotic technology.

There is far more data on the long-term survival of men receiving prostatectomies for prostate cancer than for any other treatment method. Studies show that in men having radical prostatectomy for prostate cancer, approximately 70% show no sign of a return of the cancer after ten years. This is a very good result. This is why each of the four prostate surgeons I consulted strongly encouraged me to have a prostatectomy. Their intentions were good. They wanted me to have the greatest chance of cure.

Other prostate surgeons give the same advice to men newly diagnosed with prostate cancer. This explains why over 80% of men who fit the criteria for active surveillance (Chapter 13), men who could safely watch and wait, instead opt for prostatectomy. Many doctors strongly believe that even in men with low-risk prostate cancer, the survival rate beyond 10 years favors prostatectomy. In their zeal to prevent any man from dying from prostate cancer, they recommend the surgery to virtually all their patients diagnosed with the disease. This in turn adds to massive degree of overtreatment that we see.

NEWER TECHNOLOGY CAN REDUCE MEN'S FEARS

I would add another reason for this trend. I leaned toward surgery at first because I had so many unanswered questions and so little specific information about my prostate cancer. I had to make a decision seemingly in the dark, and in that state I wanted the treatment most likely to cure me despite its serious risks to my quality of life.

Many men choose prostatectomy because they are uncomfortable with the idea of living with a potentially lethal cancer in their body while having only crude tools—PSA levels and biopsies—to monitor it. They are not comfortable with the limited information they receive about their cancer. They are uneasy about their lack of knowledge about the size, extent and possible spread of their cancer. Thus, although more than 50% of men diagnosed with prostate cancer have low-risk, localized disease, the majority of these men opt for some form of treatment, most often surgery. Is this because the doctors who diagnose them are usually surgeons?

Now, with the growing use of the DCE-MRI and to a lesser extent color Doppler ultrasound, the statistics are slowly changing. If men know their prostate cancer is localized, and that the cancer can be followed using these new tools, along with PSA levels and biopsy, far more men may choose active surveillance or a type of focal treatment such as cryotherapy, focal laser ablation, or HIFU (Steps 6-8, 10).

DOES ONE CANCER INDICATE MANY CANCERS?

Another reason urologists often recommend prostatectomy is because removing the prostate and having it examined by a pathologist has, before today's DCE-MRI, been the only way to determine exactly how much cancer the prostate actually contains. Many prostate surgeons view prostate cancer as a multifocal disease, with cancer developing simultaneously in multiple areas even if only one is located by biopsy. I spoke to four prostate surgeons and each one told me the same thing: "If you have prostate cancer in one area, you very likely have it in many other areas. Prostate cancer is a multi focal disease."

Or maybe not. A study conducted at the Cleveland Clinic and published in 2012 examined this issue. Between 2004 and 2008, 431 men were diagnosed with unilateral prostate cancer based on their biopsy findings.[1] 179 chose prostatectomy for treatment. Examination of the removed prostate glands of these 179 revealed:

In 50 men of the 179 men (28%), prostate cancer was present only on the one side of the gland. In 129 men (72%), cancer was found on both sides. In 77 of these 129 men, the cancer on the other side was small and insignificant, and did not need treatment.

In only 52 of these 129 men, the cancer on both sides of the prostate was serious and required treatment.

In summary, of the 179 men in this study with unilateral prostate cancer who underwent prostatectomy, only 29% actually needed surgery. 127 men (71%), who had no cancer or only insignificant cancer on the other side of the prostate gland, did not require surgery. They got the surgery anyway—and all of the adverse effects that often come with it.

OVERTREATMENT OR UNDERTREATMENT: A DECADES-LONG DEBATE

Experts continue to debate this ongoing issue regarding prostate cancer: Which is worse, overtreatment or undertreatment? Most surgeons believe undertreatment is worse than overtreatment, which is why they lean toward overtreatment. Undertreating prostate cancer can lead to a slow and painful death. No doctor wants this on his/her conscience. Nevertheless, many experts are no longer supportive of treatment for every prostate cancer patient without giving thought to the serious impact on a man's quality of life.

Words have never quelled the debate. Today's new technologies will. Yes, the DCE-MRI has limitations. It will not identify tiny cancers, but it will identify small and large cancers, along with unilateral and bilateral ones. It will identify whether the cancer has spread to the edge of the prostate or into other tissues. If your DCE-MRI shows a large or bilateral cancer, or that the cancer is pushing against the capsule or beyond, your decision becomes simple: surgery or radiation.

But if your prostate cancer is shown by DCE-MRI to be limited to one lobe, and this is confirmed by biopsy and by color Doppler, you have other choices. If the DCE-MRI, color Doppler and biopsy miss a cancer, then it is very small. If you follow up with ongoing surveillance including repeated PSA levels, DCE-MRI, biopsy and perhaps color Doppler ultrasound, these other potential cancers can be identified as they reveal themselves. If they are caught when they are small, focal therapy may be all that is needed.

ROBOTIC RADICAL PROSTATECTOMY

There are several techniques for removing the prostate gland surgically, but increasingly popular today is the minimally invasive, robot-assisted radical prostatectomy. This procedure has advantages in that it does not require a large incision across the lower abdomen, thereby causing less blood loss and scaring. It also allows better visualization of the prostate gland during the surgery and enables the surgeon to identify and spare some of the nerves around the prostate.

If you have a higher-grade cancer and no sign of spread beyond the prostate gland, your main treatment choices come down to surgery or radiation. In terms of long-term cure, statistics seem to slightly favor surgery. And as urologists point out, if your prostate cancer returns after surgery, you can still have radiation. But if the cancer returns after radiation, surgery is difficult because the irradiated tissue does not heal well. Today, however, focal therapies such as cryotherapy of HIFU can be used for some cases of local cancer recurrence.

THE DOWNSIDE OF PROSTATE SURGERY

Like I did, most men would strongly consider surgery if it did not come with a sobering array of side effects. The surgery itself is associated with:

• Blood loss requiring transfusion in 2% of patients
• Infection: 2%
• Blood clot in legs: 3%
• Injury to bladder or rectum: 1%
• Heart attack or heart failure: 2%
• Death: 1-2 per thousand surgeries

These statistics are not so bad considering how deep in the lower abdomen the prostate sits and that the surgery is performed mostly on men over age 50. The adverse effects following prostatectomy that worry most men are those involving bladder and sexual functioning. Even with modern robotic methods, removing the prostate always causes some damage because many delicate nerves and blood vessels run through or very close to the gland. There is no way to completely avoid these structures.

Urinary leakage may persist in 5-25% of men undergoing prostatectomy. Some men need an occasional pad, others always need them, and a few require corrective surgery. To many men, incontinence reduces quality of life immensely, even more than sexual dysfunction.

Normal sensation in genital areas and the ability to orgasm remain, but ejaculations are dry, and the quality of ejaculation and/or orgasm may change. Some men ejaculate urine. Over many months, sexual functioning can improve. Many men required erectile dysfunction drugs like Viagra, or penile injections or vacuum pumps to obtain a better erection. Shortening of the penis .25 inch to 1 inch can occur and may not improve even with therapy.

The ability to spare the neurovascular bundles is an important factor in sexual functioning after prostatectomy. If both bundles are removed, as recommended to me by Dr. Frederick, impairments are often severe and permanent.

Not all men encounter these problems after prostatectomy. I have spoken to men who bounced back with a nearly full return of urinary and sexual functioning after a few months recovery from the surgery.

Factors indicating your likelihood of normal or near normal sexual functioning after prostatectomy include your age and your sexual functioning prior to surgery. The skill and experience of the surgeon also are key. Many urologists perform only a handful of robotic radical prostatectomies a year, but it is better to have a surgeon who has done hundreds or thousands of these complex procedures. You can find surgeons with this level of experience at major medical centers or in practices that specialize in treating prostate cancer. Do not be shy about asking surgeons how many prostatectomies they have performed. Also ask about the rates of short and long-term adverse effects, and whether there is a support team to help you with post-operative problems and long-term rehabilitation of bladder or sexual functioning.

The potential adverse effects of prostatectomy are enough to cause many men to pause. However, here is the upside: This intervention has been studied more than any other current treatment method and many experts still believe it offers the best chance for cure. A study published in September 2012 in the *Journal of Urology* reported on the results of 18,209 men who underwent prostatectomy at Johns Hopkins University between 1975 and 2009. The survival rate at 10 years was 92.6%; at 20 years, 69.2%, which might sound low, except that the average age was 59 at the time of the surgery. In fact, the overall death rate from prostate cancer in the group following prostatectomy was lower than the death rate in the general male population of the same age.[2]

A 2010 study of robotic-assisted prostatectomy provided follow-up information on 1,384 men for up to seven years after surgery. At 3 years, 91% showed no sign of cancer recurrence (consistently low PSA levels); at 5 years, 86.6%; at 7 years, 81%. This study demonstrated excellent, up-to-date results on survival following robotic radical prostatectomy.[3]

As you can see, survival rates can vary from study to study. Many factors may contribute to this variability including the age of the men, the number of men in each risk category, cancer stages and Gleason scores, the general health of the men, and so on. Nevertheless, the numbers from these studies, 70-80% cure at 7-10 years, are very good.

ATTAINING THE TRIFECTA

Perhaps the number that may interest you the most is known as the *trifecta*: cure from prostate cancer, continued sexual potency, and continued urinary control. According to one study, about 62% of men obtained a trifecta in the hands of highly respected prostate surgeons at a top-notch hospital.[4] This number doesn't sound too bad. It at least gives you a decent chance at having a normal life post surgery.

At the same time, the 62% of men who regained sexual potency did not necessarily regain the same degree of functioning they had prior to surgery. In this study, sexual potency was defined as recovering enough hardness to penetrate successfully. It also counted men who required Viagra or erectile dysfunction medications to regain potency, and it included men for whom it took up to three years to regain adequate potency.

Most important in making your decision to have prostate surgery is to find a urologic surgeon you trust. In addition to having extensive experience with the technique being used, this surgeon should be willing to patiently and fully answer all your questions.

OPTIONS 2-5

RADIATION THERAPIES

The great advantage of radiation therapy is that it can treat your prostate cancer without requiring an operation. The downside is that in some cases, cancer cells survive and the cancer returns. When this happens, surgery may not be possible because the injury to the area from the radiation might impede healing. However, cryotherapy or HIFU, or a repeat course of radiation could suffice.

Another disadvantage is that as the radiation passes through surrounding tissues, it may cause damage that has an adverse impact on urinary or sexual function. Because the effects of the radiation are slow to develop, these problems may not appear for a year or more.

INTENSITY-MODULATED RADIATION THERAPY (IMRT)

IMRT is the main type of radiation therapy for prostate cancer today. It emits charged particles, primarily photons, which easily pass through the skin and intervening tissues and into the prostate gland. The beam kills the cancer cells or renders them unable to divide by damaging their DNA.

Radiation therapy technology has been steadily improving for decades. Today, radiation therapy is no longer applied with one broad beam from a single angle, but instead with narrow beams applied from many angles. Although the radiation is directed at the prostate gland, the beam also has an impact on the tissues it passes through in front and behind the prostate. This is an important consideration. However, by changing the angles by which the radiation is administered, these other tissues are minimally affected. As an example, a new machine known as Rapid Arc emits its beam from a cylinder that rotates 360 degrees around the patient, thereby minimizing the impact on other tissues.

Using CAT or MRI imaging to define exactly where the prostate is represents another recent improvement. Studies have shown that the prostate gland moves a bit when the bladder expands with urine or the rectum fills with stool. Targeting the prostate as accurately as possible is key to obtaining the best results with the fewest problems.

As the accuracy of the equipment has improved, radiotherapists have been able to increase the intensity of the radiation beam, bringing higher cure rates. This has been the most important advance in the evolution of radiation therapy.

Still, IMRT can produce impairments in sexual or urinary function. These are usually less frequent, less severe, and slower developing than with prostatectomy. In addition, as the beam passes through the wall of the rectum, burn injuries can occur. This used to be a frequent and highly vexing problem with earlier versions of radiation beam therapy. Today, the adverse effect occurs in 2-4% of patients. With IMRT, there also is a slight increase in cases of secondary bladder or rectal cancer occurring 5-10 years after radiation treatment. The increased risk is believed to be approximately 2 men per thousand per year receiving radiation.

Most forms of IMRT today require forty 45-minute sessions spread over eight weeks. Higher intensity machines such as Rapid Arc require the same number of sessions, but each session requires about 15 minutes.

STEREOTACTIC BODY RADIATION THERAPY (SBRT, CYBERKNIFE)

SBRT radiation therapy is used for many types of cancers including brain, lung, pancreas, kidney, and metastatic tumors. SBRT employs a specially designed coordination system to provide precise localization of targeted tumors. The precision of this method allows the delivery of highly potent, concentrated doses of radiation, higher than IMRT, with sub-millimeter accuracy and minimal exposure of normal tissue.

Because of the intensity of the SBRT beam, treating prostate cancer requires only five sessions, usually performed Monday through Friday. Sometimes the five sessions are staggered across two weeks, which may reduce side effects. IMRT or proton therapies usually involve smaller doses of radiation delivered over 36 to 40 weeks.

SBRT therapy begins with diagnostic scans that pinpoint the exact location of the prostate gland and cancer within it. Their movements, which shift slightly due to breathing and the subtle movements of internal organs, are plotted over time. To more accurately define these subtle changes during treatment, tiny gold seeds (fiducials) are implanted into the prostate days before treatment begins. This is done so that imaging before and during treatment can more accurately guide the SBRT. The placement of fiducials is similar to having a biopsy and also performed with imaging guidance.

The moment-to-moment precision of SBRT also allows the radiation therapist to avoid normal structures with the high-dose radiation. The SBRT beam is delivered from many different angles, thereby further concentrating the radiation into the tumor. Each SBRT session takes 30-60 minutes.

SBRT is used for single localized tumors or a few distinct tumors for many types of cancer, but with prostate cancer it is usually delivered to the entire prostate gland. SBRT can also be used for men with recurrent prostate cancer after other treatment such as prostatectomy or other forms of radiation. The benefits of SBRT versus standard IMRT or brachytherapy have been hotly debated. A 2013 article on long-term effects of SBRT showed that after five years, 97% of men undergoing SBRT for low-risk prostate cancer had no indication of cancer recurrence based on PSA monitoring. Moreover, 91% of men with intermediate-risk cancer and 74% of men with high-risk prostate cancer had no indication of cancer recurrence. These are pretty good numbers and comparable to other forms of radiation therapy. Adverse events with SBRT involving bladder or rectum were similar to those with IMRT. Impotence occurred in only 25%.[1] The most commonly reported side effect with SBRT is mild fatigue for a week following treatment. Some men have reported intense, immediate adverse effects with SBRT, probably due to the high intensity of the beam used.

BRACHYTHERAPY

This form of radiation therapy involves implanting small radioactive seeds into the prostate gland. The seeds are the size of tiny grains of rice, a few millimeters in diameter. They are placed via a needle inserted through the perineum (the area between the scrotum and the anus) into the prostate gland. The advantage of brachytherapy is that a high dose of radiation can be delivered directly into the prostate gland, thereby causing less injury to surrounding structures than occurs using IMRT. Another advantage of brachytherapy is that the procedure is accomplished in one outpatient surgery rather than a lengthy series of visits. Some experts believe that overall, brachytherapy is the most effective form of radiation for prostate cancer.

Brachytherapy can affect bladder, sexual or bowel functioning. Approximately 10% of men develop urinary symptoms, including a constant urge to urinate, or slow or painful urination. These adverse effects can last for months.

PROTON BEAM RADIATION THERAPY

Unlike IMRT that irradiates with photon particles, proton beam radiation employs protons to kill prostate cancer cells. Theoretically, the advantage of proton beam therapy is that it only releases its energy when it reaches its target. Other tissues through which the proton beam passes are not affected, thereby greatly reducing adverse affects. The big question is whether proton therapy has perfected the ability to release its energy in the prostate and not elsewhere. Recent articles appearing in medical journals state that proton beam therapy is effective for prostate cancer, but it has not been shown to be superior to IMRT or brachytherapy.[1]

The newest version of proton beam therapy, also known as intensity modulated proton therapy, utilizes a narrow "pencil beam," which allows greater control over radiation doses and shorter treatment times. This approach has less impact on surrounding tissues, thereby reducing the incidence of side effects. A study of men under age 61 found a low degree of impact on sexual functioning following treatment for prostate cancer with proton beam therapy. Proponents of proton beam therapy also claim that the therapy has little impact on bladder control.

However, another large review of Medicare patients with prostate cancer who underwent proton beam therapy showed a slightly higher rate of rectal bleeding than others who received standard IMRT.

A bigger problem is that in August 2013, Blue Shield of California announced it would no longer cover claims for proton therapy. Why? Because proton therapy costs tens of thousands of dollars more than other types of radiation therapy but, as the Los Angeles Times article puts it, "a slew of studies have found that proton therapy doesn't yield better results than older, cheaper alternatives."[1A] "Proton beam is really the perfect example of all that is wrong with our healthcare system," said Cary Gross, a researcher at the Yale School of Medicine who recently compared outcomes for 30,000 Medicare patients who received proton beam or standard radiation. "The rush to adopt proton beam is far outpacing the amount of evidence to support its use."[1A] The study also found that one year after treatment, side effects were not less than with other radiation therapies.

Another insurer, Cigna, has said it considers proton beam to be equal but not superior to standard radiation. As a result, Cigna does not consider proton therapy as medically necessary in many cases. Aetna also lists proton therapy for prostate cancer as not medically necessary and nor proven more effective than other radiation therapies. On the bright side, Medicare continues to pay for proton therapy for prostate cancer and, I believe, so do secondary insurers for people who have Medicare. How Obamacare will handle proton therapy is unknown at this time. Therefore, always check with your insurer as part of your planning for proton radiation therapy.

Notice, no one is claiming that proton therapy is less effective than other radiation approaches, and some men who have had it speak very highly of it. Tens of thousands of men have been treated for prostate cancer with proton beam radiation, and you can find hundreds of glowing testimonials on the Internet about the effectiveness of proton therapy.

Like IMRT, proton therapy requires daily visits for 6-8 weeks. Today, proton therapy is available at a handful of medical centers in the

U.S.:

- CA: Loma Linda University, Loma Linda
- CA: Scripps Proton Therapy Center, San Diego
- FL: University of Florida, Jacksonville
- IL: ProCure Proton Center, Warrenville (near Chicago)
- IN: Indiana University, Bloomington
- MA: Massachusetts General Hospital, Boston
- NJ: ProCure Proton Center, Somerset
- OK: ProCure Cancer Center, Oklahoma City
- PA: University of Pennsylvania, Philadelphia
- TX: M.D. Anderson Cancer Center, Houston

Proton therapy centers are being developed in several other cities including Baltimore (University of Maryland), Atlanta (Emory University), and at the Mayo Clinic in Minnesota and Phoenix, AZ.

RADIATION FOR PROSTATE CANCER: HOW EFFECTIVE?

In terms of long-term survival from prostate cancer, many doctors believe that recent advances in radiation therapy have brought this approach to a level of equality with prostatectomy. Moreover, adverse effects from today's radiation therapies are less frequent and less severe than those with prostatectomy. The men in my group reflect a spectrum of treatment interventions, but the greatest number received IMRT. Several years post-treatment, they remain in remission and have had fewer adverse effects so far than those who chose prostatectomy. These men remain bullish on radiation treatment for aggressive prostate cancer. Then again, many of the most serious adverse effects from radiation therapy can appear years after treatment ended, so the final chapter for these men who chose radiation remains unfinished.

In an article published in August 2012, the survival rate after ten years among 2,658 men with prostate cancer was 89% following prostatectomy, 87% following EBRT (external beam radiation therapy, an early version of IMRT), and 83% with brachytherapy.[2] The study also focused on how many men developed a secondary malignancy such as bladder, rectal or other pelvic cancer. At 10 years, 3% of men who had a prostatectomy had developed a secondary malignancy, 2% following radiation, and 4% following brachytherapy. This study suggests that concerns about increased incidences of secondary pelvic cancer after IMRT are unwarranted. On a broader note, the ten year survival with these therapies are similar, with prostatectomy and IMRT being virtually equal and holding a slight edge over brachytherapy.

Other studies have indicated somewhat lower success rates with IMRT. A 2007 article revealed a 5 year cancer free rate of 74-86% following IMRT. This study used a lower radiation intensity than employed today.[3]

A 2011 study in the journal *Cancer* reported the outcomes of men with prostate cancer treated with IMRT. Ten years after treatment, 100% of men with low-risk cancer showed no indication of metastases, and in 81% of these men PSA levels remained low. The ten-year numbers for men with intermediate-risk cancer were 94% without metastases and 78% had low PSA levels. For men with high-risk cancer the numbers were 90% without metastases and 62% with low PSA levels.[4]

Overall, these results suggest that if you require treatment for your prostate cancer, you should include radiation therapy among your treatment considerations. This is not to say that radiation therapy always goes smoothly. During the months of uncertainty about my case, I decided to pursue radiation treatment. I interviewed four radiation doctors, all of whom seemed first rate. I was diligent about letting them know about my history of neuropathies, severe nerve injuries I have in my legs. These neuropathies had developed for no apparent reason in 1995 and were so painful and untreatable, they rendered me bedridden for five years and disabled for another five. I finally developed a treatment regimen that worked, and I am doing fine now. However, when I talk to new doctors, I make sure to inform them about the condition.

The first radiation session went well, but after the second session, my severe neuropathies flared badly, causing pain and difficulty walking. I had told this radiologist about my neuropathies, but apparently he forgot during his treatment planning. For my part, I neglected to do adequate research. The medical literature has a half dozen reports about radiation causing neuropathies.[5-12] My radiation oncologist could have designed the radiation beam to avoid the nerves as they exited the spinal cord and descended down my legs, but he didn't. Even good doctors make mistakes. We both erred in failing to recognize that the very intense beam of Rapid Arc would be risky in a person with highly sensitive neuropathies, and that a more gentle approach such as IMRT might be a better fit. After the incident, I spoke to another radiologist who suggested shaping the beam properly and eliminating the risk, but I was not going to chance it. As it was, it took weeks for me to get the neuropathies back under control.

I hope you will not have to deal with such complications, but if you do, you are not alone. In medicine, many cases have divergent results, unexpected reactions or other idiosyncrasies. At times, only a minority of cases match the examples in the textbooks. If you have any medical conditions or sensitivities, be sure to inform your doctors and gather your own information from books, articles, or on the Internet.

I should not have assumed my radiation doctor had broad knowledge in this area. Perhaps he had never before run into this problem with a patient receiving radiation therapy. I should have been more circumspect and reviewed the medical literature myself. So, I repeat: Do not assume your doctors know how to deal with your individual conditions and circumstances.

B: FOCAL THERAPIES

For decades, the medical approach to treating prostate cancer has been based on the premise that if prostate cancer is found on biopsy, it likely exists in many parts of the prostate gland. This explains why doctors have so often recommended radical treatments that entail removing the entire prostate gland or irradiating it, even to men with low-grade, Gleason 6 cancer. This is why overtreatment has been and continues to be so rampant.

Yet as Dr. Dan Sperling, M.D., writes, "Radical treatments themselves pose inherent risks: post-treatment urinary, sexual and bowel morbidities (side effects). The recent debate over routine PSA screening of healthy men stems from a well-placed concern that men with a rising PSA are rushed into invasive, blind needle biopsies that entail risks of infection, false negative, and under-staging. A positive biopsy triggers an intense period of decision-making with whole-gland treatment often being the physician's first recommendation."[1]

In the past, we did not have the technological capability to differentiate the men who actually needed whole prostate treatment (prostatectomy or radiation) from the men who didn't. Before DCE-MRI and color Doppler ultrasound, a man who declined radical treatment was making a risky wager. Today, the availability of the DCE-MRI has reversed the risk. In my case, when the MRI and color Doppler ultrasound both showed a modest-sized, solitary tumor in a safe area of my prostate gland, a tumor that was not near any vital structures, it became much easier for me to consider a less aggressive approach.

Quietly, more men have been opting for focal treatment of their prostate cancer. The treatment modalities most often used are cryotherapy or high intensity focused ultrasound (HIFU). As the prostate DCE-MRI has become available, men have chosen these techniques with greater confidence. A newer method, MRI-guided focal laser ablation (destruction by intense heat), is also available now. It too is applied in a targeted manner with DCE-MRI guidance during the procedure.

So today, many experts as well as patients are now asking: Why treat the whole prostate if only one part of it has evidence of cancer? Proponents of focal therapy compare it to a lumpectomy that many women choose for localized, low-grade breast cancer.

The main advantage of focal therapy is that while destroying the cancerous lesion in the prostate, healthy tissue including the nerve bundles that control sexual and bladder functioning can be spared. For example, the most vexing adverse effect with HIFU of the whole prostate gland is urinary stricture (severe narrowing of the urethra), but this problem can be avoided when HIFU is used for focal treatment.

In a recent article in the *Wall Street Journal*, Dr. Gary Onik, who performs cryotherapy (a freezing technique) in Orlando, Florida, said, "Focal cryosurgery offers a middle ground between watchful waiting and more aggressive therapies. Let's ablate the cancers we know about, and then do watchful waiting. Meanwhile, the minimally invasive procedure can be repeated if the cancers reoccur."[2]

If a new tumor arises in the prostate after treatment a focal therapy, the same method can usually be used to remove it.

OPTION 6

CRYOTHERAPY

Cryotherapy (cryoablation) is a non surgical method of destroying prostate cancer cells by freezing them. The use of cryotherapy began fifty years ago and methods have improved greatly in recent years. Today, cryotherapy is performed using 3D and Doppler ultrasound in fusion with DCE-MRI imaging, allowing accurate identification and measurement of areas of prostate cancer.

Cryotherapy involves no cutting and little blood loss. The treatment is done through the wall of the rectum and takes a couple of hours. Cryotherapy does not involve any radiation, and it may be repeated if the cancer returns locally. It may also be used for salvage treatment of recurrent prostate cancer following prostatectomy or radiation. Radiation therapy can also be done if cryotherapy fails.

The most vexing adverse effect from full prostate cryotherapy is erectile dysfunction. This side effect occurred very often with early forms of full prostate cryotherapy. The shift from total to focal cryotherapy has reduced this problem greatly. Urinary incontinence and injury to the rectal wall are infrequent adverse effects.

RESULTS FROM STUDIES

Studies of cryotherapy have demonstrated improving results as the emphasis has shifted from full-prostate treatment to focal treatment and as techniques and imaging methods have advanced. The emphasis for this approach has also shifted away from high-risk prostate cancer to low and intermediate risk cases.

For example, in a study by Bahn et al., focal cryotherapy assisted by color Doppler ultrasound was conducted with 31 men with unilateral prostate cancer.[1] Six years later, 93% of men showed no elevation in their low PSA levels, and 96% had negative biopsies. Sexual potency was maintained by 48% of the men, and another 41% regained potency with medication. In other words, adequate potency was obtained in 89% of the men, a far better number than with prostatectomy or radiation therapy.

FINDING A DOCTOR WHO PERFORMS CRYOTHERAPY

A Google search for "cryotherapy prostate cancer" reveals a wealth of information about cryotherapy and its practitioners. I know two doctors who perform cryotherapy here in Southern California. Both are highly rated and have published studies of cryotherapy in medical journals:

Duke Bahn MD: Prostate Institute of America, Ventura, CA 93003, 888-234-0004, pioa.org.

Osamu Ukimura M.D., Ph.D.: Keck Medical Center of the University of Southern California, 800-872-2273, doctorsofusc.com.

I met Dr. Ukimura last year at the Center for Image-Guided Surgery and Focal Therapies at the University of Southern California Keck Medical Center. He told me that he and Dr. Bahn have continued to refine the technology used with cryotherapy, further improving outcomes and reducing incidences of adverse effects. They now use MRI-ultrasound fusion technology for performing cryotherapy.

You can find other practitioners of cryotherapy in a Google search of "cryotherapy prostate cancer" and your city. My expectation is that cryotherapy will continue to increase in popularity as more men with prostate cancer consider focal treatment.

OPTION 7

FOCAL LASER ABLATION (FLA)

Initially developed to treat brain tumors, MRI-guided focal laser ablation is now approved for treating cancers in soft tissues including spinal cord, muscle, kidney, liver and prostate. Laser treatment uses light energy delivered by a probe positioned into the core of the tumor. As the intensity of light increases, the temperature of the probe rises and destroys the cancer cells. The doctor will also burn a margin of normal prostate tissue surrounding the tumor to make sure all of the cancer cells are destroyed.

The DCE-MRI imaging plays a key role in ensuring that the laser treatment is delivered to the proper area. The laser probe is inserted into the man's body via the perineum (between the testicles and anus) and directed by the doctor between other pelvic structures and toward the prostate. Once in the prostate gland, the laser probe is threaded using MRI guidance into the proper area of the gland and then into the tumor. The entire focal laser ablation (FLA) procedure takes 2 to 4 hours, and most of it is used for accurately positioning the probe. Once there, the intense heat of the laser destroys the tumor in about 10-15 minutes. As this occurs, the changes of the cancerous tissue from the laser's intense heat can be seen on the MRI images. This helps guide the doctor to deliver the correct amount and duration of laser-generated heat is administered.

Today, there are a handful of practitioners in the U.S. who perform focal laser ablation for prostate cancer. One of them is Dr. Dan Sperling, who states that with MRI guidance, he is able to identify prostate cancer tumors as small as 4 millimeters and then destroy them with FLA.[1]

Compared to HIFU and cryotherapy, laser therapy seems a much simpler and direct approach. Dr. Sperling told me, "Focused laser ablation of prostate cancer isn't much different than performing a biopsy." Except that a biopsy only requires taking twelve or so pieces of prostate tissue, which is accomplished in about 10-15 minutes. You can see Sperling's Youtube video at http://www.youtube.com/watch?v=lX1d--Dx56A.

Dr. Scott Eggener, a urologic oncologist at the University of Chicago Medical Center, calls focused laser ablation "the equivalent to women with breast cancer having a lumpectomy."[2]

Dr. Sperling states, "Focal therapy is rapidly presenting itself as a middle ground, energetically sought by patients and cautiously championed by a minority of clinicians. Advances in imaging technology now make it possible to clearly detect smaller and smaller tumors, and advances in targeted ablation enable effective ablation of even a small focus of disease."[1]

FLA with MRI guidance is also available under the direction of Sharif Nour, M.D., at Emory Healthcare, Atlanta, GA, and so does the group at Desert Medical Imaging, Indian Wells, CA. The University of Texas Medical Branch also offers FLA. Its chairman of radiology, Eric Walser M.D., has been performing this procedure for three years. "The problem is, most men who test positive, even if the risk is one in 1,000 of dying of prostate cancer, still just want to get it out of there," says Dr. Walser. "Our approach pairs the most advanced MRI imaging to identify cancer-suspicious areas in the prostate and the most advanced laser technology to remove them, with virtually no risk of impotence or incontinence."

OPTION 8

HIGH INTENSITY FOCUSED ULTRASOUND (HIFU)

Robotic high intensity focused ultrasound, or HIFU, is currently being tested in FDA approved clinical trials. The procedure is already being used in Canada, Europe and South America, and we will likely see this technology in the U.S. in a few years. Today, several U.S. urologists will evaluate you in their offices, then perform your HIFU treatment in Bermuda, Mexico or Europe.

HIFU destroys cancerous prostate cells by heating them to nearly 212 degrees Fahrenheit while leaving nearby structures unharmed. HIFU is not a form of radiation therapy, so it doesn't have any of the adverse effects of radiation on surrounding tissues. HIFU is performed with a probe through the rectum and into the prostate, so no cutting is involved, little blood loss occurs, collateral damage is minimal, and recovery is relatively quick. Indeed, HIFU is performed as an outpatient procedure. Treatment typically takes two to three hours.

HIFU can be tailored to the needs of each patient. It can be used to destroy the entire prostate gland, one of its lobes, or one specific area of the prostate. HIFU can be performed on all stages of prostate cancer and on all Gleason scores. It can also be used as a salvage treatment when cancer returns after prostatectomy, radiation, prior HIFU or other types of treatment.

ADVERSE EFFECTS WITH HIFU

As with robotic prostatectomy, the HIFU doctor can see the area being treated, thereby avoiding vital structures such as the seminal vesicles and neurovascular bundles. This capability allows for lower rates of adverse effects. After HIFU, men will require a urinary catheter for 2-4 weeks. Incontinence or urinary retention (unable to urinate) occurs in a small percentage of men.

The most common significant adverse effect with HIFU is urinary stricture, a scarring of the urethra through which urine flows. Stricture occurs in approximately 25% of men after HIFU prostatectomy. This happens much less frequently in men receiving single lobe or focal HIFU, as do most other adverse effects.

Sexual dysfunctions and bladder control difficulties can occur with whole gland HIFU as often as with surgery or radiation treatment. When used for focal treatment, HIFU causes fewer of these problems.

Total prostate HIFU cannot be performed on men whose prostate size is over 40 cc. In men with larger prostates, medication is often prescribed to shrink the prostate gland before proceeding with HIFU treatment.

MORE LONG-TERM STUDIES NEEDED

A major downside of HIFU is the lack of results from long-term studies. One of the most recent publications describes a study of 157 men with various degrees of prostate cancer treated with HIFU. After 5-year follow-up, 66% of low-risk men lacked any sign of cancer recurrence, as did 40% of intermediate-risk and 21% of high-risk men. Men without any sign of cancer spread were 74%, 46%, and 29% respectively. These results do not compare with those following prostatectomy or radiation therapy. The authors commented: "HIFU treatment does not provide effective oncologic outcomes even in low-risk patients with prostate cancer, as well as in intermediate or high risk groups."[1]

Another study showed a cancer-free rate of 69% seven years after HIFU treatment.[2] This rate does not equal the results following prostatectomy or radiation therapy today.

At the same time, these results should be considered preliminary because they reflect men treated with HIFU in the early and mid 2000s when clinicians had limited experience with a still developing technology. Today, many doctors have implemented the use of DCE-MRI guidance in performing HIFU, which should improve results with this therapy.

YOU CAN CONTACT DOCTORS
WHO PERFORM HIFU

You have the opportunity to ask about these results and other questions with doctors who perform HIFU. Because they are seeking subjects for FDA-approved clinical studies for patients seeking HIFU off shore, some practitioners of HIFU will speak to you directly. I spoke to three doctors, and each seemed experienced and highly knowledgeable. In alphabetical order I spoke to:

- Douglas Chinn M.D.: Chinn Urology, Arcadia, CA (near LA), 626-574-7111, chinnurology.com.
- Stephen Scionti M.D.: Scionti Prostate Center of Boston, Milton, MA, 02186, 866-866-8967, drscionti.com
- Ronald Wheeler M.D.: PanAm HIFU, Sarasota, FL 34239, 877-766-8400, panamhifu.com.

Other U.S. doctors perform HIFU, and you can find them with a basic Google search of "HIFU prostate cancer." Because HIFU is not available in the U.S., getting treatment can be costly. Having HIFU in Bermuda, Mexico or Europe can cost up to $20,000. HIFU is available in Canada. For example, the Cleveland Clinic in Toronto offers HIFU. The contact information is: Maple Leaf HIFU, Ancaster, Ontario, Canada, L9G 4V5, 877-370-4438, hifu.ca/index.htm.

My first urologist, Dr. Summers, disdained HIFU, calling it something like "doing surgery with a hot curling iron." However, I was interested in this new technology and spent considerable time reading about it. In addition to the three doctors I mentioned above, I also talked to two HIFU patients who spoke highly of their experiences.

As it becomes available in the U.S. and the price begins to drop, HIFU may become more popular. The use of HIFU will likely increase as the emerging diagnostic technology such as the DCE-MRI makes focal treatment a popular choice for localized prostate cancer. A small study published in 2011 using HIFU for focal therapy in 20 men with low or intermediate-risk prostate cancer showed that persistent adverse effects were fewer than seen with prostatectomy or radiation therapy. One year after HIFU treatment, 95% of men continued to have erections sufficient for vaginal penetration; 90% of men were continent without urinary leakage or the need for pads.[3]

C. NON-INVASIVE THERAPIES

OPTION 9

MEDICATION THERAPY FOR PROSTATE CANCER

A boy's prostate gland is tiny. With puberty and the first surges of testosterone from the testes, the prostate gland begins to enlarge until it is the size of a walnut. About seventy years ago, Dr. Charles Huggins discovered that removal of the testes markedly slowed prostate cancer progression. And so it became widely accepted that reducing testosterone in the body hindered prostate cancer growth.

Medications that reduce testosterone's impact on prostate cancer are known as "androgen deprivation therapy" or ADT. Occasionally it is called TIP for "testosterone inhibiting pharmaceuticals." ADT drugs block the stimulating effect of testosterone on prostate cancer cells. Generally, an ADT approach is preferred before chemotherapy because it is less toxic and generally more effective initially.

Today, ADT therapy is used most often at the later stages of treatment for aggressive cancers, after prostatectomy or radiation therapy, sometimes after metastases have already spread outside the prostate gland. It is often overlooked for men with low or intermediate-risk prostate cancer. Back when my doctors told me I had intermediate-risk prostate cancer, not one of them mentioned this frequently effective approach. Yet this approach has many advantages when used for intermediate-risk disease. The main benefit of ADT is that it can allow men to avoid surgery or radiation for years or decades, and sometimes altogether.

ADT: HOW IT WORKS

Treatment with ADT most often involves drugs that provide three types of synergistic, anti-testosterone effects. A drug frequently used for turning off testosterone production in the testes is Lupron (leuprorelin, Eligard). The drug is administered as a monthly or long-acting quarterly injection.

Another group does not lower testosterone per se, but instead blocks the androgen receptor at which testosterone impacts prostate cells and prostate cancer cells, thereby reducing testosterone's effect on the cells. The best-known androgen receptor blockers are Casodex (bicalutamide) and Nilandron (nilutamide).

The third group, the 5-alpha-reductase inhibitors such as Avodart (dutasteride) and Proscar (finasteride), block the chemical conversion of testosterone to dihydrotestosterone, which is 5 times more potent. By doing so, these drugs greatly reduce the potency of the testosterone reaching the prostate cancer cells.

When ADT is used for advanced prostate cancer, its effectiveness usually lasts 3-6 years, at which point the cancer may develop resistance to the drugs' effects. For men with early, intermediate-risk prostate cancer, the effect can extend 10 years or more.

ADT's impact can be rapid and dramatic. Within 8 months, many men with newly diagnosed prostate cancer see drops in their PSA levels to far below 1 ng/ml, often as low as 0.05 ng/ml, meaning that the activity level of the prostate cancer has been reduced to near zero.

CASE REPORTS ON ADT

Mark Scholz, M.D., co-author of the excellent *Invasion of the Prostate Snatchers* and a pioneer in ADT for intermediate-risk prostate cancer and sometimes in concert with active surveillance for low-risk disease, writes "over the years we have seen hundreds of men with excellent responses to ADT." Here are three of the many cases he has described.[1]

A man with a PSA of 34 was found to have Gleason 6 prostate cancer. After starting ADT, in two months his PSA was 0.3. He discontinued ADT two years later after a biopsy showed no residual cancer. His testosterone levels returned to normal a year after that. He has remained off ADT for 15 years while continuing with active surveillance. So far he has not needed any further treatment.

In 1997, a 78 year-old man had a PSA level of 33. Digital rectal exam revealed multiple palpable areas suggestive of prostate cancer. Biopsy determined he was intermediate-risk.

He began ADT therapy, which reduced his PSA rapidly. The man continued ADT therapy for 18 months then discontinued. His testosterone level recovered quickly. Multiple color Doppler ultrasound tests have revealed stable areas of prostate cancer. He has never required additional ADT. In 2008, at age 90, his PSA level remained at a very low 0.6 ng/ml.

Also in 1997, a 64 year-old man with PSA 12 was found to have an intermediate grade prostate cancer in one area of his prostate gland and low-grade cancer in two other areas. He began ADT treatment, and five months later his PSA was too low to measurable. He discontinued ADT therapy. Six years later a biopsy showed a recurrence of his intermediate-grade cancer. ADT was restarted, his PSA dropped again and one year later his biopsy was clear. ADT was discontinued. As of 2009, his condition remained stable.

Although the typical ADT triad is comprised drugs such as of Proscar, Casodex, and Lupron, Ralph Blum, the second author of *Invasion of the Prostate Snatchers*, did it differently. He agreed to take Lupron only. However, Blum also took Casodex for a few days before starting Lupron. The Casodex blocked the brief flare of testosterone that can cause unpleasant side effects when initiating treatment with Lupron. Today, doctors often prescribe ADT by starting with one or two drugs at a time rather than all three simultaneously. They then add a third when the first drug loses effectiveness.

Blum began Lupron in December 2002, and 4 weeks later his PSA had dropped from 18.3 to 10.3 ng/ml. Seven months later, his PSA was 0.125. He discontinued Lupron for 4 months. When his PSA level crept back to 1.05, he restarted Lupron. He went off and on Lupron for many more years, ultimately deciding to have radiation therapy. The delay his ADT afforded was worthwhile, because during his years on ADT the accuracy and effectiveness of radiation treatment improved greatly.

Many doctors start ADT with Avodart, which they favor over Proscar. If it becomes necessary, Casodex may be added when Avodart's effect wanes. Third comes Lupron, if needed. Drugs, dosages and regimens can vary considerably between different doctors.

HOW DOES ADT RATE OVERALL?

A study of ADT treatment in men with newly diagnosed prostate cancer revealed the following results. The study included 73 men, average age 67, with an average PSA of 9, and a majority of men with DRE findings suggestive of prostate cancer. Most of the men were intermediate-risk and some were high-risk. All of the men took ADT for 9 months or longer. At 12 years follow-up, 21 (29%) of the men never required any further treatment. Twenty-four men (33%) required periodic ADT to keep PSA levels below 5. Other men ultimately elected to have invasive treatment (surgery or radiation). And 3 men had died 3, 8 and 11 years after starting ADT treatment.[2]

The main finding of the study was that 29% of the men with intermediate or high-risk prostate cancer never needed any further treatment after their initial course of ADT, and another 33% were maintained with intermittent ADT treatment. In other words, 45 men (62%) never needed surgery or radiation or other invasive treatment.

In all cases, testosterone levels gradually returned to normal after discontinuation of ADT. With today's superior monitoring abilities using DCE-MRI and/or color Doppler ultrasound for following the progression of prostate cancer, the results with men on ADT will likely be even better.

Over time, it has become clear that for men with intermediate-risk prostate cancer, ADT is another option to consider.

THE DOWNSIDE OF ADT

The results with ADT for prostate cancer are impressive, and all it takes is a few pills a day or a monthly or quarterly shot. But the fact is that if you have intermediate-risk prostate cancer, there are no easy treatment choices. Most men who have intermediate-risk prostate cancer require treatment. The choices are prostatectomy, one of the many forms of radiation therapy, one of the focal therapies (if the cancer is localized)—or ADT.

Taking pills is certainly easier than invasive treatment. However, as you might imagine, taking pills that inhibit testosterone has many undesirable effects on the male body and mind. First and foremost, ADT markedly reduces libido. Your sex drive may drop to nearly zero.

Erectile dysfunction drugs like Viagra can help produce an erection, but many men don't bother because they have no desire for sex. Blum writes that he couldn't imagine not having any desire for sex, but when he was on ADT, even though Viagra worked for him, "I couldn't dredge up enough desire even to want sex." Not every man experiences this side effect to this degree, but many do.

Other ADT side effects include loss of muscle mass, fatigue, weight gain, night sweats and daytime hot flashes, breast growth (often not reversible), osteoporosis (bone loss), joint pains, and increased emotionality. Some men say they can minimize the muscle loss, fatigue and weight gain by regular exercise with weights and a healthy diet. If hot flashes and sweats are bothersome, other medicines can block this adverse effect. Yet other side effects can be more difficult to reduce.

These problems seem monumental to most men, but before rejecting this approach, consider the adverse effects with the other options. Surgery: 50 percent impotence and 8% incontinence, which are often permanent; all of the other adverse effects and risks of the surgery; and return of cancer in 25%. Radiation IMRT: 35% impotence, 2% rectal burn, 2% urethral inflammation, and return of cancer in 25-30%.

The fact is, the adverse effects of ADT can vary greatly from man to man. For this reason, ADT should be started on a trial basis. For example, Lupron can be effective for many men, while others are greatly affected by fatigue or severe hot flashes. A good example of this is if you and your doctor decide to try Lupron first, start with the monthly injection rather than the extended-release three-month injection. If severe side effects hit, you know the side effects will subside within a month rather than having to wait three months.

Many doctors today prefer to start ADT with Avodart because adverse effects are somewhat less. Avodart blocks dihydrotestosterone, the primary and most potent stimulus of prostate cancer among a man's hormones. When this drug's benefit wanes, doctors often add or replace Avodart with Casodex. Today, Lupron is often held for last.

On the positive side for ADT, some men with intermediate-risk disease only need it once and others intermittently. Some men can go off ADT for months or years at a time. Testosterone levels typically rise again, sex drive and normal sexual functioning return in most men, but not all. Long-term loss of normal sexual functioning has been reported with Proscar (finasteride) and Avodart (dutasteride) lasting months or years after the drug has been stopped. More on this in Step 12.

NEWER ADT DRUGS FOR ADVANCED PROSTATE CANCER

In 2011 and 2012, two new drugs, Zytiga (abiraterone) and Xtandi (enzalutamide), were approved by the FDA for the treatment of "castration-resistant prostate cancer," meaning that standard ADT treatments no longer worked. The term originated from a time when the only form of ADT was castration, which greatly lowered testosterone levels. When castration no longer worked, or in modern times standard ADT no longer works, the prostate cancer is called castration resistant. Because Xtandi and Zytiga are extremely potent blockers of testosterone, they can have many side effects. Be sure to ask about this if your doctor recommends either of them for your prostate cancer. For example, Xtandi can increase the risk of seizures.

Xtandi was purposefully designed to overcome the androgen receptor resistance that occurs with many men on long-term ADT. Xtandi works by blocking the androgen receptor of prostate cancer cells approximately five times more tightly than Casodex (bicalutamide). In addition, resistance to Xtandi may develop more slowly than with standard ADT drugs. In studies, Xtandi was shown to markedly reduce PSA levels and to extend life significantly more than placebo in men with castration resistant, metastatic prostate cancer.

Zytiga is also used as a treatment for castration resistant prostate cancer that is metastatic. The drug blocks the production of androgen in both the testes, adrenal glands, and the tumor itself. Studies have shown that Zytiga significantly slows the progression of metastatic prostate cancer, delays the time when men had to start chemotherapy, and modestly improves survival times. Because of its many adverse effects, Zytiga is taken with prednisone, a form of cortisone.

CHEMOTHERAPY

If you need to speak to a doctor about chemotherapy for your prostate cancer, you have high-risk disease and possibly metastatic disease. You want to be sure the doctor is knowledgeable and highly experienced. Some urologists specialize in the chemotherapy of high-risk prostate cancer, but the majority of urologists do not. The same can be said about oncologists, who are doctors specializing in the treatment of cancer. Most oncologists treat many types of cancer.

My recommendation is to find an oncologist who specializes in treating prostate cancer, or at least an oncologist whose practice includes a lot of cases of prostate cancer. Don't hesitate to ask the doctor about his/her experience with your type and degree of prostate cancer, as well as their experience in prescribing the drugs I have discussed in this chapter and chemotherapeutic agents.

Also, be sure to read Step 11 on the new genetic tests that are available today for improving the accuracy of biopsy interpretation and for enhancing cancer aggressiveness grading. Most of all, if you may need chemotherapy, read about the new genetic tests to identify the most effective chemotherapy drugs based on the genetic profile of each man's prostate cancer.

OPTION 10

ACTIVE SURVEILLANCE

*A*ctive surveillance is the treatment method chosen by many men with low or, sometimes, intermediate-risk prostate cancer. Previously, an approach called *watchful waiting* was used with some men with low-risk disease. Many men did well on this program including Eddie Carrillo, a Los Angeles contractor who was diagnosed with prostate cancer at age 52.

According to an article in the *New York Times*, Mr. Carrillo's primary care doctor and urologist both recommended prostatectomy. Mr. Carrillo happened to hear about watchful waiting and decided to monitor his cancer. Now, 15 years later, Carrillo remains healthy at age 67. "I wasn't ready to do the operation right away," Mr. Carrillo said. "I have two uncles with prostate cancer, and I have quite a few friends who have had their prostates taken out. The discomfort level and what they went through afterward, I didn't think that was the way I wanted to go."[1]

Watchful waiting actually began in the 1970s. The idea was that prostate cancer was a slow growing disease and people didn't die from it. This proved dead wrong in too many cases. So, with the advent of PSA testing in 1989, an opposite approach took hold. If your PSA level was high, a biopsy was done. If the biopsy showed cancer, aggressive treatment—prostatectomy or radiation—was recommended. The view was that if a biopsy showed cancer, the likelihood was that there was more cancer in the prostate, and radical treatment was needed to prevent death. The problem with this approach was that prostatectomy and radiation caused injury to surrounding tissues, often permanently impaired men's sexual or bladder functioning, and in about 25% didn't cure the cancer anyway.

The only other alternative was watchful waiting. The problem with this approach was that it really did what it said—watched and waited—sometimes waiting too long before initiating treatment.

A MODERN PERSPECTIVE

Through the 1990s and into the 2000s, it has become increasingly clear that many men, as they age beyond fifty, develop small areas of prostate cancer. The percentage of men having these small prostate cancers generally reflects their age group. For example, around 70% of men at age 70 have these small cancers in their prostate. Yet, because men's prostate glands often enlarge as they age, their PSA levels also climb. With the findings of an elevated PSA and a biopsy positive for cancer, these are the men who have been sent for prostatectomy or radiation—often unnecessarily.

A key shift has begun in the recognition that these non-threatening cancers are usually Gleason 6, low-grade and non-threatening. Dr. Laurence Klotz explains,

Active surveillance was an attempt to grapple with this by saying, okay, we know that guys who have bad prostate cancer need treatment, and benefit from it. And that's been clearly shown in randomized trials. But the patients dying of prostate cancer tend to have higher grade (Gleason) cancer. So maybe we can take the ones who have low-grade cancer, just manage them conservatively, and keep a close eye on them because some may develop something worse. So we started doing that [in studies] around 1996, more than 15 years ago. At the time, it was considered very experimental, and patients had to sign an informed consent form that they were going on a clinical trial. Yet patients flocked to this approach, because word was getting out that there were problems with the outcome of surgery and radiation in terms of quality of life.[2]

Now, after more than fifteen years of study, it has been demonstrated that hardly any of these men with small, Gleason 6 prostate cancers die. Less than 2% die over 10 years. Dr. Klotz adds,

The vast majority of men who are found to have these little bits of low-grade cancer have absolutely no threat to their life, and can be managed with conservative treatment.

Many other experts agree. Leonard Marks M.D., Professor of Urology, UCLA, states, "Prostate cancer is so prevalent, many men during their lifetime will be diagnosed with prostate cancer. Unlike a lot of cancers, breast, lung, colon, there are some prostate cancers that just sit there. They don't kill you. So even though these are, technically, cancers, they're not lethal cancers."[2A]

ACTIVE SURVEILLANCE TODAY

Today's active surveillance is different than the watchful waiting of the 1990s and 2000s. Active surveillance involves frequent testing, keeping a close eye on a man's cancer with repeated PSA levels and an occasional biopsy. To my mind, these two tools are not enough to assure men that if there cancer grows larger or shows signs of spreading, intervention will be mobilized quickly enough. This is why I initially decided to have surgery. But if you add the new diagnostic methods—DCE-MRI and color Doppler ultrasound—active surveillance can be highly effective. When I obtained these tests, I decided to forego surgery and take the active surveillance route.

WHO IS A CANDIDATE FOR ACTIVE SURVEILLANCE?

In 2007, the first national conference was held on active surveillance for prostate cancer. A consensus protocol was developed to define the men appropriate for active surveillance.

- Normal DRE (digital rectal exam)
- Gleason score of 6 or less
- 2 positive biopsy cores or fewer
- No biopsy cores comprised of 50% cancer cells or more
- PSA level less than 10

Men who select active surveillance must be committed to working closely with their doctor. PSA levels should be drawn every three months for a year, then every 6 months. Digital rectal exams need to be done every 6 months at first. Biopsies have also been part of the protocol, but these may be less necessary today for men who are getting DCE-MRI or color Doppler ultrasound testing. None of these tests are 100% accurate, yet taken together they can provide an early warning of worrisome changes in your prostate cancer.

You may have noticed that my findings did not fit all of the criteria for active surveillance. I fit only three of the five factors: Gleason level 6; DRE normal; no biopsy cores greater than 50% cancer. However, my PSA levels were 15 and 13, well above the ceiling of 10 to be categorized as low-risk. Yet, with my large prostate and history of prostate infections, the PSA levels might not have been as bad as they seemed. PSA levels are accurate only about 75% of the time. In men like me, who have complicating factors, PSA levels are less reliable.

Also, my biopsy revealed 4 (of 14) cores with prostate cancer, which are more than the 1 or 2 positive biopsy cores allowed under the usual definition of low-risk prostate cancer.

As you can see, decision making may be simple or complicated, depending on your findings. I discuss this further in the next chapter, *Weighing the Evidence and Making a Decision.*

WHEN TO CONSIDER TREATMENT

If any of the tests above suggest worsening of your prostate cancer, consideration must be given to the possibility of active treatment. Changes for the worse include:

- Increasing PSA levels
- Abnormal digital rectal exam
- Increase in cancer size or signs of spread on DCE-MRI or color Doppler ultrasound
- Biopsy cores with a Gleason score of 7 or more
- 3 or more biopsy cores with cancer

WHY MEN DO NOT CHOOSE ACTIVE SURVEILLANCE: "THE CUT-IT-OUT-NOW" SYNDROME

Approximately 240,000 men in the U.S. will be diagnosed with prostate cancer in 2014. About half have early stage disease that will probably never harm them. These men fit the criteria for active surveillance, yet 90% of them will elect prostatectomy or radiation therapy. Why is this?

"Men have a strong belief that if they are diagnosed with cancer, they will die from the cancer if it's left untreated, and a belief that treatment will cure them," said Dr. Timothy Wilt.[3]

The diagnosis of cancer produces so much anxiety, many men want to get rid of the cancer *right now*, no matter the risks to their quality of life afterward. The rate of heart attacks and suicide doubles in men who are told they have prostate cancer. Other men do their homework, weigh the benefits and risks, do not act rashly, yet still decide they will sleep better knowing the cancer has been removed. Others are pressured by family members, who are scared by the term "cancer." Other men listen to only one voice, their urologist, a surgeon. Others are not told about the new diagnostic methods and multiple, focal treatment options. They have followed the traditional path: PSA, biopsy, surgery or radiation.

A recent study showed that when men with newly diagnosed prostate cancer discussed treatment with only their urologist, only 10% choose active surveillance. This is only one fifth of the men who actually match the criteria for active surveillance. In contrast, when men with newly diagnosed prostate cancer met with a team of experts including a surgeon, radiologist, and MRI specialist, about 40% of the men eligible for active surveillance choose it. More information gave the men more choices.

IS ACTIVE SURVEILLANCE REALLY AS SAFE AS SURGERY OR RADIATION?

An important study on the use of active surveillance for prostate cancer was published in July 2012 in the *New England Journal of Medicine*. The study consisted of 731 men with prostate cancer who, between 1994 and 2002, were treated with either prostatectomy or watchful waiting. 364 men received prostatectomy, and of these 21 (6%) ultimately died of prostate cancer. 367 men received watchful waiting, with 31 (9%) ultimately dying from their cancer. Overall, surgery for prostate cancer produced 3% fewer deaths than watchful waiting. In terms of preventing death from prostate cancer, prostatectomy was slightly superior.[4]

But at what cost? During the thirty days after prostate surgery, complications caused one death, two cases of blood clots in the legs, two more in the lungs, one case of renal failure, one stroke, blood transfusions in six men, six others requiring urinary catheters more than thirty days, and 10 cases requiring further corrective surgery. Problems with bladder control from dribbling to complete loss of urinary control occurred in 49 men with surgery versus 18 men with watchful waiting. 81% of men who had surgery developed erectile dysfunction, compared with 44% in the watchful waiting group.

Overall, prostatectomy slightly reduced the risk of death or metastases from prostate cancer in the high and medium risk groups, but at the cost of many serious adverse effects that clearly impaired men's quality-of-life. These adverse effects were experienced by men after surgery no matter whether they were high, intermediate or low-risk. Yet, in the low-risk group the study found no benefit whatsoever from surgery in reducing the risk of death or metastases in comparison to watchful waiting.

This study was the first to clearly define the advantages of watchful waiting versus prostatectomy in men with low-risk prostate cancer. "I think this is game changing," said Dr. Leonard Marks, a urology professor at UCLA. "What this study does is call attention to the fact that there are a lot of prostate cancers that are diagnosed today that are not dangerous."[3]

Also, this study used watchful waiting. Today, with the availability of the DCE-MRI, active surveillance will demonstrate even greater protection than watchful waiting did in men with low-risk disease.

I am not saying that active surveillance is always preferable to aggressive treatments such as prostatectomy or full gland radiation. These therapies play a crucial role for men with higher Gleason levels, abnormal DRE or other worrisome findings. The key is to accurately differentiate which men need which treatment. And for men with low-risk cancer who are not comfortable knowing they harbor cancer in their prostates, the focal therapies can provide safer, less injurious ways to remove the cancer without causing lifelong impairments in bladder and sexual functioning.

The key to all of this is obtaining an accurate diagnosis that defines the type and grade of cancer you have and pinpoints where it is located. PSA, DRE, DCE-MRI (and if available, color Doppler ultrasound) are all key players in accomplishing a level of diagnostic accuracy that has not been possible previously.

"We just finished collecting data on 520 men undergoing active surveillance up to 10 years," Dr. Duke Bahn said in an October 2013 interview. "During that ten years' time, we found that about 30% of men needed some treatment because [color Doppler] ultrasound clearly showed disease progression. Increased blood flow in the known cancerous lesion was the first sign of the cancer progression. So 30% of men in this cohort ended up having proper loco-regional treatment. We did not have any patients who developed metastases or who died. No one got into trouble. The point here is that 70% of men are doing just fine up to ten years. This result is similar to other published data. Certainly, proper patient selection was the key to this favorable outcome."[5]

NO FRINGE IDEA

Active surveillance is no fringe idea. In 2011, the National Institutes of Health, the leading authority on health issues in the U.S., formally validated the approach:

Active surveillance has emerged as a viable option that should be offered to patients with low-risk prostate cancer. More than 100,000 men a year diagnosed with prostate cancer in the United States are candidates for this approach.[6]

You may find you are one of these men if you have done your homework and have obtained the tests I recommend.

OPTION 11

ALPHARADIN FOR BONE METASTASES

The first big breakthrough of 2013 was the Carbon-11 PET/CT Scan, which I discussed in Step 8. The second big breakthrough was alpharadin, which the FDA approved for widespread use on March 15, 2013. Unfortunately, at that time Alpharadin's manufacturers, Bayer Pharmaceuticals and Algeta ASA (Norway), took the opportunity to change the drug's name to Xofigo. Too bad. Alpharadin was one of the best medication names I've ever heard. Catchy and easy to remember, "alpharadin" also reflected the character of the drug itself, radium-223, and its activity, emitting alpha particles to destroy cancer that has metastasized to bone. What a great all-in-one name! On the other hand, Xofigo sounds like some kind of fancy condom. What were they thinking?

No matter. Alpharadin is the first drug of its kind, a drug that fixes specifically to calcium and other minerals in bone that allows it to deliver radiation directly to cancer metastases.[1] Because radium-223 is chemically similar to calcium, it is readily attaches itself like a magnet to bone. The alpha particles are highly lethal to cancer cells harbored there. Alpharadin is intended for men who have been treated with surgery or radiation, or medication therapy to lower testosterone levels, or chemotherapy. It is not designed for men whose prostate cancer has spread to other organs of the body. Alpharadin will also be used for other types of cancer that spread to bone. One likely use will be for women with metastatic bone cancer.

GREATER EFFECTIVENESS, FEWER SIDE EFFECTS

Cancer experts agree that alpharadin represents a therapeutic step forward. Commenting on recent scientific reports, medical oncologist Jean-Charles Soria, MD, PhD, stated, "I think that [radium-223 chloride] will become a major player in prostate cancer management." Michael Baumann, MD, professor of radiation oncology at the University of Technology in Dresden, Germany, added, "This is a very important finding. It is certainly practice changing."[2]

Alpharadin's properties allow for a marked reduction in adverse effects compared to earlier isotope therapies that target cancer metastases in bone. Strontium 89, which emits beta particles that cause greater peripheral damage, has been used infrequently because of its many adverse effects, especially suppression of bone marrow cells. Samarium 153, also a beta emitter, causes fewer problems but has still been withheld except for very advanced metastatic bone disease.

Unlike the above therapies, alpha particles have a very limited range, only 2-10 cells deep, thereby causing much less injury to surrounding healthy tissues. The half-life (how long it takes for half of the substance to leave the body) of alpharadin is just 11 days, which makes it ideal as a targeted, limited, radioactive cancer therapy. Residual alpharadin is rapidly dispatched to the intestinal tract and eliminated.

Most importantly, alpharadin is the only direct radioactive agent demonstrating improvement in overall survival time in studies of men with prostate cancer bone metastases. In the Symptomatic Prostate Cancer (ALSYMPCA) trial, men receiving alpharadin demonstrated a median survival time of 14.9 months vs. 11.3 months for men receiving placebo.[3] This large trial involved 921 subjects at over 100 treatment facilities in 19 countries. Treatment consisted of monthly intravenous infusions of alpharadin or placebo over six months. The trial is ongoing but no longer recruiting subjects. The results were so encouraging that the FDA sought a priority review and granted early approval.

Although an increase of 3.6 months in longevity may seem small, it is statistically significant. Moreover, many men experienced greater benefit, and it should be remembered that all of the subjects had very advanced prostate cancer. Now that alpharadin has been approved, doctors will likely use it earlier in men exhibiting bone metastases. Such metastases occur frequently in men with advanced prostate cancer, especially in those with prostate cancer resistant to testosterone blocking therapies ("castration resistant prostate cancer"). The most common side effects in the study were nausea, vomiting, diarrhea, and swelling of the legs, ankles or feet. Other adverse effects included reduced red and white blood cell and platelet blood counts.

OPTION 12

TOO GOOD TO BE TRUE?
PROSCAR (FINASTERIDE) TO
PREVENT PROSTATE CANCER

If you have already been diagnosed with prostate cancer, this approach does not apply. However, for men who are concerned about getting prostate cancer or who have a higher risk (African-American or a blood relative who's had prostate cancer), a study published in August 2013, "Drug Cuts Prostate Cancer Risk," announced that the drug finasteride (Proscar) significantly reduces the risk of getting prostate cancer.[1] But before you sign on, be sure to read the fine print.

Having analyzed thousands of medical studies, this one, "Long-Term Survival of Participants in the Prostate Cancer Prevention Trial," published in the *New England Journal of Medicine*, wins a prize as one of the most misleading and alarming studies I've seen.[1A] The study was big, 18,880 men over 18 years, costing $73 million. Back in 2003, when the first phase of the study was published, I saw many flaws in the approach it suggested.[2] I wasn't alone. Dr. Peter Scardino, one of the most prominent urologists in the U.S. and chairman of the department of urology at Memorial Sloan-Kettering Cancer Center in NYC, wrote in an accompanying editorial. "Should finasteride now be recommended to men in order to lower their risk of prostate cancer? Several disturbing findings in the report argue that it should not."[3]

A BAD STUDY RECOMMENDS A
BAD DEAL FOR MEN

Think of it this way. If we gave 10 million men finasteride, it would reduce their risk of prostate cancer by 38%. Sounds good, but at what cost? Finasteride blocks the conversion of testosterone into its more active derivative, dihydrotestosterone, which is ten times more powerful than testosterone itself. Blocking this conversion can have profound effects on men. Thus, common side effects include reduced libido (10%), abnormal ejaculation (7.2%), impotence (18.5%), breast swelling (2.2%; which is sometimes painful), and abnormal sexual functioning (2.5%).[4] These numbers are from the manufacturer of finasteride and the FDA, so they are credible, but be aware that manufacturer's numbers often underestimate the true frequency of side effects.

Worse, these symptoms do not always recede after the drug is discontinued. They can last for months or years. It is not believed to be a common problem, but nor does it seem to be rare. The condition has a name: Post-Finasteride Syndrome. It is believed to occur infrequently, but who really knows? Is 'infrequent' 1 in 10 men, 1 in 100, 1 in 1,000? From my research on the drug industry, it appears that drug companies do not really want to find answers to these types of questions, nor do they want the attention such answers would attract. Many doctors who treat sexual disorders are aware of PFS. So is the FDA. For more information, go to http://www.pfsfoundation.org/contact/.

The same problems have also been reported with Avodart (dutasteride), which is in the same family as, and often used instead of, finasteride. A study in the 2011 Journal of Sexual Medicine confirms it.[5] Most men who take these drugs experience some of these side effects, but according to Abdulmaged Traish, M.D., lead author of the study, "some experience it more drastically than others." Dr. Traish added that in a small percentage of cases, "It is a life sentence. No sex. No desire. Potential depression."[6]

So, of the 10 million men to whom we gave finasteride, the incidence of prostate cancer would probably drop from 16% to 11%. That's good. But *all* of the 10 million men would be subject to getting the side effects from blocking testosterone. Plus, 8.4 million of these men would never have gotten prostate cancer in the first place. Still interested, fellas?

FINSATERIDE REDUCES LOW-RISK CANCERS BUT MAY INCREASE HIGH-RISK ONES

The second reason finasteride for preventing prostate cancer is a terrible idea is that it only lowers your risk of the low-grade forms of prostate cancer. These are the types that rarely harm. So reducing the incidence of low-risk prostate cancer from 16% to 11%, as discussed above, may be good but it isn't really as big a deal as it sounds. Unless, of course, with today's backward methods, your doctor rushes you to biopsy, then surgery or radiation. If you have read this far in *Prostate Cancer Breakthroughs 2014*, you know how to avoid overtreatment.

The study also found that finasteride was associated with a small increase in the incidence of high-risk cancer. If this is true, it is another good reason to trash this idea. Further analysis suggests that this finding might be a statistical artifact due to the design of the study. Nevertheless, the chief researcher of the study, Dr. Ian Thompson, felt the need to address it during his press conference. "Even if there is a higher risk of high-grade cancer, it doesn't appear to have an impact on how long a man lives, and that's reassuring."[7] No, it isn't reassuring. If the drug truly increases the occurrence of high-risk prostate cancer, however slightly, it means more prostatectomies or radiation therapy. These in turn mean more sexual and bladder dysfunctions and reduced quality of life.

I doubt many men will opt to take finasteride every day for the rest of their lives to prevent prostate cancer of which they have only a 16% chance of getting, especially since the drug can markedly reduce their sex drive, performance and pleasure. In addition, the drug only protects men from low-grade cancer, the kind that can be handled today with focal therapy or active surveillance.

It is difficult to understand why this study was ever funded. Or why it made the national news. It just goes to show that in today's rush-rush world, members of the media often draw their reports from the press releases they are given. Few take the time or have the training to read a scientific article and sort the true breakthroughs from the busts.

SECTION 3

WEIGHING THE EVIDENCE
AND
MAKING A DECISION

Step 9

WHAT DOES YOUR DATA SAY?

Making a decision about treating your prostate cancer is not always simple. Even if you and other men have the very same test results, you may get a different recommendation from your doctor than a man with similar test results gets from his doctor. Even with similar input from doctors, different men may choose different treatments. This is why it is important to organize your test results and then consider the appropriate treatment choices.

When you have finished your tests, list all of the results together and see how they add up.

TABLE 13.1: YOUR TEST RESULTS

Spread your test results and extenuating factors,
and see how the results add up.

TEST	RESULTS	RISK LEVEL
PSA levels:		
Positive biopsy cores:		
T Grade:		
Gleason Score:		
Color Doppler ultrasound:		
DCE-MRI findings:		
Genetic Tests (if done)		
Carbon-11 PET/CT Scan (if done)		
Extenuating factors (if any):		

The next table shows how my data looked.

TABLE 13.2: MY TEST RESULTS

TEST	RESULTS	RISK LEVEL
PSA levels:	15.3, 13.4	Intermediate
Positive biopsy cores:	4 positive for cancer	Intermediate
Biopsy grade:	T1c	Low
Gleason score:	6	Low
Color Doppler ultrasound:	Small solitary lesion, no spread	Low
DCE-MRI findings:	Small solitary lesion, no spread	Low
Genetic Tests (if done)		
Carbon-11 PET/CT Scan (if done)		

My Extenuating Factors:

#1: 75cc prostate volume inflated PSA results, making PSA more accurately 11-12 ng/ml, slightly above the low-risk ceiling of 10.

#2: 4 biopsy cores showing cancer was above the 2 required for active surveillance; yet Scholz and also Katz allow 3 of 12 cores to be positive, and because of one of my cores was only 1% cancer, Scholz felt my biopsy cores fit the low-risk category. Other experts disagree, stating that 2 positive cores or fewer are required for low-risk status.[1,2]

Consider one more factor when analyzing your findings: Which test results are most important?

Looking at my results, I considered the Gleason score of 6, indicating a less aggressive cancer, the most important finding. The DCE-MRI and the confirmatory findings with the color Doppler ultrasound were the next most important. These tests showed and confirmed that I have a small, solitary tumor in a relatively safe area of my prostate gland, not near any vital structures or showing any indication of spread outside of the prostate. Putting it all together over five months, my treatment choice became much easier: active surveillance.

It is important to remember that no single test is enough to decide where you stand or what to do. None of the tests for prostate cancer are 100% accurate, but rather are 75-90% reliable. How do you deal with this imprecision? As Dr. Scardino of the Sloan Kettering Cancer Center put it, "I don't rely just on the digital rectal exam, the PSA, the biopsy results or the MRI. But if we put all that information together, we can get a pretty good idea of what's going on."[3] In fact, this isn't some new method of evaluation and diagnosis. The basic medical approach to diagnosing any patient is: history, physical exam, laboratory tests, and other tests. Every medical student learns this. So why the problem in obtaining a DCE-MRI or color Doppler ultrasound? If the test doesn't jive with the other findings, you and your doctor can always ignore it.

Your case may be *typical*, in which the all of the findings fit nicely into one risk category. Or it may be *atypical* like mine, with some results fitting one category, and other results fitting another. Atypical cases are common in medicine, sometimes so common that they outnumber the textbook cases. *This is why it is important to obtain all of the tests you can and as many opinions as you need.*

If your findings are similar to mine, doctors stuck in today's outdated model will almost invariably recommend surgery or radiation. They will look at your PSA levels and biopsy cores and make their recommendation to you, just as they recommended prostatectomy or radiation for me.

The problem with the current model is that it has not caught up with the new, 21st century technologies. Medical guidelines are determined based on long-term studies that are replicated and confirmed. For example, a long-term study of the DCE-MRI can take many years, and to have the results confirmed by other studies takes additional time. Then the urology associations have to review the data and draw up new guidelines. All of this is unlikely to happen before 2015 and perhaps not until 2020.

Meanwhile, conservative urologists, which include most urologists today, will remain slow to embrace the new tests, and insurance companies may not pay for them yet. Hadn't Dr. Summers, my urologist, who did a good job in determining that I had prostate cancer, discounted the utility of a DCE-MRI? Hadn't he refused to order this test even though I offered to obtain it elsewhere and pay for it myself?

Your urologist may act the same way. Remember, urologists are most often surgeons, so they will have a particular point of view. Be prepared for this. If you don't agree with the opinion, stay calm, thank the doctor for his/her opinion, and seek a second opinion.

ASSESSING THE DOCTOR YOU CHOOSE

The surgeons and radiologists I consulted were highly recommended, intelligent and experienced people. They were truly concerned about me and really wanted to help. Yet to my mind, they were strictly following the 20th century model: high PSA and positive biopsy, go directly to prostatectomy or radiation.

At first, until I learned otherwise, that's how I looked at my case too. As I mentioned earlier, I actually started Rapid Arc IMRT radiation in April 2012, but the beam was improperly designed for the severe nerve injures (neuropathies) in my legs. The photon beam hit the nerves descending from my spine, aggravating my condition. My setback was acute and serious, and I had to immediately discontinue treatment. This experience was a blessing in disguise, because it shocked me into thinking twice and twice again about the risks of treatment and whether, with my DCE-MRI findings, I needed treatment at all.

Unlike the surgeons and radiologists, Dr. Scholz paid attention to the DCE-MRI report and performed the color Doppler ultrasound that confirmed the MRI results. This willingness to use up-to-date technology is one reason I like him. Scholz said the cancer was small and located in a relatively safe area of the prostate gland. Because of this, he said, there was a 90% likelihood that it would never bother me. Scholz is one of the top prostate cancer oncologists in the country. He is one of

134

the top experts on active surveillance and has evaluated hundreds of cases like mine. I could not have chosen a more appropriate doctor for my case than Scholz.

Yet I had to consider, he could still be wrong. I like Scholz and look forward to my next appointment with him. At the same time, all doctors have their biases and blind spots. By the very nature of his writings, Scholz clearly leans away from prostatectomy and toward active surveillance. I had to consider this fact too.

If your doctor recommends surgery or radiation based solely on your PSA and biopsy findings, which many doctors still do, you should take pause and get a second opinion, if possible from a doctor who is not a surgeon and not in the same health care system. You should ask your doctor about the DCE-MRI for the prostate gland. Remember, this is different than the standard MRIs used today. Has your doctor heard of the DCE-MRI? Would he or she consider giving you an order for the test? If not, is the doctor agreeable to your obtaining another opinion from an expert who knows about the DCE-MRI, color Doppler ultrasound, genetically-based tests, and other recent breakthroughs?

Even though I am Gleason 6 and have a localized tumor, I still meet doctors today who recommend prostate surgery or radiation. My DCE-MRI and color Doppler ultrasound findings do not alter their views. They are not even aware of the genetic tests for when there is doubt. You may need to consult with several doctors. Some men create their own medical team consisting of their primary doctor, urologist, prostate surgeon, radiation specialist, and prostate cancer oncologist.

If you are Gleason 7, for example, you want to have a doctor who knows the difference between Gleason 3 + 4 versus Gleason 4 + 3. Remember, the numbers represent the levels of aggressiveness. Gleason 3 + 4 indicates that the most prevalent cancer in your prostate is Gleason 3, whereas with Gleason 4 plus 3 the most prevalent cancer is the more aggressive 4. Some doctors recommend very different treatments for these two types of Gleason 7 cancer. You want a doctor who understands these distinctions and can discuss them with you.

Perhaps your findings are severe, with a very high PSA level or a Gleason score of 8 or above. You are high-risk, so the tests I am recommending should be performed as part of your diagnostic work-up. A DCE-MRI is important to delineate the extent of your cancer. Is it on one side or both? Is it encroaching on the prostate capsule? Has it spread elsewhere? The new Carbon-11 PET/CT scan is key for determining whether there are metastases. All of these details are essential because the treatment of a Gleason 8 to 10 prostate cancer can be quite different depending on whether the cancer has grown beyond the capsule and into surrounding tissues or has metastasized to distant sites.

WHAT DOES THE SCIENCE SAY?

You may also find it helpful to read the reports of studies that are relevant to your type of prostate cancer. For example, the 2012 study in the *New England Journal of Medicine* was key to my choosing active surveillance as my current treatment. As discussed in the chapter on active surveillance (Option 10), this study unequivocally showed that for men with low-risk prostate cancer, watchful waiting was just about as effective in 10-year survival as prostatectomy.[4] This finding does not mean that all men with prostate cancer should choose active surveillance, but it is a reasonable consideration for men with low-risk disease. My view is that if watchful waiting was effective in this study, today's active surveillance will be more so. Watchful waiting was limited to PSAs and biopsies, whereas my active surveillance program also includes follow-up color Doppler ultrasound and DCE-MRI testing, and perhaps in late 2013 genetic testing to hopefully confirm my cancer's low level of aggressiveness. These tests are a big improvement over yesterday's watchful waiting, because they can improve the speed and accuracy of identifying any worsening of my prostate cancer.

The study mentioned above also found that of the 364 men who underwent prostatectomy, a large majority of those with low-risk cancer had no other cancers in their prostate glands or only small, insignificant ones. A conservative doctor would say yes, that's true, but the men with significant bilateral cancer were saved. I agree, but rather than doing prostatectomies on all of these men, why not use the DCE-MRI to sort them out first? Dr. Scardino writes, "The level of treatment should match the risk posed by the cancer."[3] This is why the diagnostic tests, especially the DCE-MRI, are so important. Unless you get this and all other important testing, how can you and your doctor know the risk posed by your cancer?

I also found it helpful to watch the DVDs of experts who lectured at the monthly support group meetings I could not attend in person.

These DVDs are available from the Informed Prostate Cancer Support Group at ipcsg.org. Click on "Purchase DVDs." You can also find various presentations by experts on prostate cancer by searching Google for "prostate cancer youtube."

The newer tests have an important impact on me in another way. By using them as part of my active surveillance, I no longer feel that I am flying blind. Psychologically, this is a big relief.

WHY LOW-RISK MEN CHOOSE HIGH-RISK TREATMENT

It is unfortunate that today, a large majority of men who are low-risk and who would be good candidates for active surveillance or focal therapy nevertheless choose to undergo prostatectomy or radiation treatment. Both of these therapies can cause serious, permanent adverse effects that greatly reduce men's quality of life. The unnecessary damage occurs so often—about 80,000 men each year who get aggressive treatment for low-risk disease—the medical associations have recommend we stop PSA testing. In essence, they are saying, "Better to not identify prostate cancer with PSA testing than to identify prostate cancer and over treat it." But what about the 25,000 men whose lives are saved each year by PSA testing? Is it right for us to abandon them.

Why do these men with a low-risk prostate cancer choose more intensive and risky treatments than they need? One reason is that they feel acutely vulnerable. Being given the diagnosis of "cancer" has that effect on many men, and the instinct is to take immediate action. With the old model, with only PSA levels and biopsy results to guide them, these men feel very much in the dark about their prostate cancer. As I learned all too well, it is extremely stressful not to know how big your cancer is, where it is located, whether it is in one or both lobes, and whether it has spread. It is difficult to live with the knowledge you have a cancer inside of you that may kill you, yet know so little about it.

I expect that as doctors begin implementing the DCE-MRI and genetic testing as diagnostic tools, a much larger percentage of men will select active surveillance. In an article in the New York Times on genetic testing, Dr. Eric A. Klein of the Cleveland Clinic said, "Even if we can only convince 15 to 20 percent of men that we have enough confidence that they don't need to be treated, that will be a big step forward."[5] The availability of DCE-MRI (or multiparametric MRI) testing is also expanding. I listed eight centers in the 2013 edition of *Prostate Cancer Breakthroughs*. In this new edition, I list 20.

Focal treatment is also gaining greater favor. Prostatectomy and radiation will remain important therapies for some men, and the new diagnostic tests will improve their results by sorting prostate cancer patients properly before radical treatment is chosen hastily. When these developments become routine, prostate cancer treatment will have truly entered the 21st century.

MY CURRENT GAME PLAN

My plan in June 2012 was follow the active surveillance protocol to the letter. I obtained another PSA level in May 2012, and it was 12.4; I repeated it again in August, and it was 13.0. These levels were slightly lower than the previous 15.3 and 13.4. The difference between them is negligible. Basically, my PSA levels were holding steady. As long as they did not escalate, I was content.

In the back of my mind, I sometimes thought about having the cancerous nodule in my prostate gland treated focally. Surgery and radiation are performed only on the full prostate. And while HIFU and cryotherapy can also be used to treat the whole prostate, they are more frequently used for focal treatment, as is focal laser ablation. Still, even these focal therapies had risks I would rather have avoided. Instead, I preferred to play for time, hoping I am in the 70% of men in active surveillance who never need treatment.

Then, in October 2012, my PSA nearly doubled again, shooting up to 26. I was shocked. I contacted my doctor. He told me that with prostate cancer, PSA levels rarely shoot up like that. PSAs rise more gradually. The most likely cause was an infection or inflammation. Did I have any signs of these? I had no signs of infection, but I do have an inflammatory disorder that had been causing more symptoms lately.

Dr. Scholz suggested I take Cipro or Levaquin, the best antibiotics for prostate infections, for three weeks. He didn't know that I had written one of the first medical journal papers on the severe and long-lasting side effects that these drugs cause,[6] albeit rarely, and that I have added more recent information on this problem at my website, MedicationSense.com. I asked him if we could wait a little longer as I increased my anti-inflammatory therapy. The next PSA was 22, and a month latter it was back to 14. I also got another color Doppler ultrasound test followed by a DCE-MRI, the 3.0 Tesla type at UCLA. The results were the same as in January 2012. All was again quiet.

Today I continue to watch as new studies are published and new advances in technology emerge. The odds are 30% that I will need intervention someday, so I am keeping my eyes open. Perhaps I will get one of the genetic tests, but I have not decided.

Hopefully, I will never need intervention. Yet every time I have another PSA level drawn, I worry whether that it will jump up again. So I keep doing my homework while preparing myself for any possibility. Once you have had prostate cancer, or any cancer, no matter what treatment approach you chose, you are always on active surveillance for the rest of your life.

STEP 10

30 QUESTIONS TO ASK YOUR DOCTORS

Prepare for your meetings with your doctors. Bring the following list of questions and circle the ones you want to ask. The questions should be relevant to the purpose of the meeting. If you try to ask all 30 questions at one meeting, you will wear your doctor out. Doctors are human after all, so be fair and respectful of the doctor's time. Too many questions may provoke frustration.

Bring a notepad. If you have a wife, significant other, or close family member or friend, consider bringing one of them. Studies have shown that people remember only a fraction of what doctors tell them. A notepad and a companion can really help.

Bring an open mind. Different doctors have different experiences and points of view. It is certainly reasonable to ask follow-up questions or request the basis of a doctor's opinion or recommendation, but remain calm and respectful. If you disagree with the doctor's approach or recommendations, seek a second opinion rather than arguing with the doctor. If possible, the second opinion should be with a doctor from a different group or institution. I say this because many groups and institutions have created their protocols that all of their doctors follow. In order to obtain a truly independent second opinion, you may need a doctor not associated with your first doctor's organization. If this is not possible, get a second opinion from a different type of doctor such as an oncologist in your healthcare system.

Also bring information you have gathered from books or the Internet. Doctors are sometimes resistant to Internet information, but a good doctor will be open to data from respected sources such as medical institutions, medical journal articles, the National Institutes of Health (NIH), the American Urologic Association, books written by experts and supported by studies and references.

Most of all, try to remain positive. The survival rate of men after ten years with prostate cancer is 95%.

1. Is my PSA level normal or elevated?
2. If it is elevated, how elevated? What might it mean?
3. Other than cancer, are there other possible causes of my high PSA level?
4. Can we repeat the PSA test before initiating other tests?
5. Can you do the digital rectal exam and the ultrasound now to accurately measure my prostate size?
6. If my prostate gland is enlarged, how much might it affect the PSA results?
7. If my PSA levels are both significantly elevated, what does this mean? What is the next step? Antibiotics? Biopsy?
8. Can you refer me to a good prostate cancer support group? (Remember, you can access all of the lectures from my support group, Informed Prostate Cancer Support Group ipcsg.org).
9. If a biopsy is needed, can we arrange a targeted one instead of a random (blind) one?
10. Can we obtain a DCE-MRI test to determine whether a tumor may exist before doing the biopsy?
11. Do you perform a color Doppler ultrasound for prostate cancer? If not, do you know of any doctors who do?
12. If a tumor is seen, can you use the DCE-MRI or color Doppler ultrasound to perform a targeted biopsy?
13. If the biopsy is negative, should we consider one of the new genetic tests to confirm whether the biopsy interpretation?
14. If my biopsy is positive for cancer, what Gleason score do I have and what does it mean?
15. Should I get a second opinion on my biopsy cores and Gleason score?
16. Should we consider genetic testing to confirm the grade and aggressiveness of my prostate cancer?
17. Is there any sign that the cancer has spread?
18. For men with high-risk cancer: Would a Carbon-11 PET/CT Scan be helpful in determining whether I have metastases.
19. What treatment do you suggest for me? If prostatectomy or radiation therapy, can I speak to the surgeon or radiologist?
20. I have read about other types of radiation therapy: SBRT, brachytherapy, proton therapy. Can you tell me about them?

21. What are the risks of treatment failure and of adverse effects with these aggressive treatments?
22. Are there alternatives to surgery or radiation therapy I should consider? What about androgen deprivation therapy (ADT)?
23. Do you think that focal therapy might be appropriate for my prostate cancer?
24. Have you heard of cryotherapy, focal laser ablation, or high intensity focused ultrasound (HIFU)? Might one of these be worth considering for my cancer?
25. Am I a candidate for active surveillance?
26. Even though you have advised active surveillance, I am uncomfortable with the thought of cancer within my prostate gland. What other choices do I have?
27. I have intermediate-risk prostate cancer. Many treatments have been recommended: prostatectomy, radiation, ADT—which one do you recommend?
28. I have high-risk cancer with signs of metastases: what do you advise?
29. Am I a candidate for alpharadin?
30. What about genetic tests for selecting the most effective chemotherapy medications?

Question 31 is, Are you with the right doctor? You have a serious disease. You have a right to ask questions and receive full answers. If your doctor is unable or unwilling to answer your questions, find another doctor who will.

SECTION 4

CONCLUSION

I spoke to Jonathan this morning. He is a friend of a friend. His recent PSA results were 8.5 ng/ml and on retest 9.2, significantly elevated numbers. His doctor recommended a biopsy, the typical blind biopsy that I told you about in Step 2. I told Jonathan to look for a doctor who performs color Doppler ultrasound testing with which a targeted biopsy could be performed.

"I know all about blind and targeted biopsies," Jonathan replied. "My recently deceased wife had cancer and needed a liver biopsy. The initial scan was unclear, so the doctors went ahead and did a blind biopsy. They missed the cancer areas, subjecting my wife to a lot of unnecessary and prolonged pain. When they repeated the scan, it showed exactly where the suspected metastases were. A targeted biopsy was done and provided what we needed to know. "

Prostate biopsies are something you do not want to do twice, yet they are frequently repeated in men with suspected prostate cancer because the first blind biopsy found nothing. We cannot blame doctors for wanting to be sure not to miss a cancer, but this should not be an issue today. As this book has described, there are better ways.

"My doctor told me that if my biopsy is positive for cancer, the next step would be prostatectomy," Jonathan told me. "What do you think?"

I urged Jonathan to do a Google search for "color Doppler prostate cancer Baltimore," his city. In the event he was unable to find a color Doppler specialist nearby, and because Jonathan often travels west for business, I also gave him the names of doctors around Los Angeles who perform targeted biopsies using the color Doppler ultrasound (Drs. Mark Scholz, Richard Lam, Douglass Chinn, Osamu Ukimura, Duke Bahn; see Step 6).

Jonathan's targeted biopsy found cancer, Grade 8, high risk. He is now finishing a full course of IMRT radiation therapy.

THE MOST IMPORTANT FACTOR:
AN ACCURATE DIAGNOSIS

If you ask Richard, a 65 year-old with prostate cancer, what is the most important part of evaluating prostate cancer, he answers without hesitation, "The accuracy of the diagnosis." He says this because several years ago, his PSA went over 6 ng/ml, and cores from a blind biopsy revealed a Gleason 6 cancer on one side of his prostate gland. Repeated PSA results remained steady, so Richard chose active surveillance, although his urologist recommended prostatectomy.

A year later he consulted with Dr. Duke Bahn, who performed a color Doppler ultrasound and targeted biopsy. The more accurate targeted biopsy showed bilateral prostate cancer with a Gleason 7 cancer in one lobe and Gleason 8 in the other.

His cancer had advanced to the point that Richard was no longer a candidate for prostatectomy, and instead radiation and androgen deprivation (ADT) therapy were recommended. ADT is no picnic. As I explained in Option 9, reducing a man's testosterone level to almost zero can lead to osteoporosis, hot flashes, depression, breast enlargement, diabetes, obesity and high blood pressure, not to mention diminished libido and impaired sexual functioning. Now Richard wonders if his original blind biopsy was accurate. Was active surveillance the correct initial treatment? Apparently not. Should he have chosen prostatectomy instead? If he had obtained the color Doppler ultrasound sooner or a DCE-MRI, would his treatment choices have been more appropriate? Could he have avoided ADT? Would his long-term prospects have been better?

"One thing that I feel certain about is the need for complete diagnostic testing including the new modalities that are now available," Richard told me. "Too much testing is better than too little, because prostate cancer can be an insidious disease and difficult to diagnose accurately. Many cases like mine deviate from the established norms. The more you learn about your cancer, the better your chances of successful treatment."

My view is that a DCE-MRI and/or color Doppler ultrasound should be done as part of the diagnostic workup of *all* men who might have prostate cancer. It should be used just as we use standard MRIs today in so many other areas of medicine to help determine diagnoses

148

before resorting to invasive methods. A biopsy is an invasive method, so it should be targeted, not blind.

And when a biopsy reveals prostate cancer, genetic testing should be considered to confirm that the Gleason grade is correct. Genetic testing also be helpful to ensure that a negative biopsy is truly negative. The only questions about genetic testing are whether it is reliable and affordable.

A BETTER APPROACH FOR DIAGNOSING PROSTATE CANCER

1. Elevated PSA level, then...
2. Digital rectal exam and ultrasound to measure prostate size, then...
3. If there is a possible prostate infection, treat with antibiotics, then...
4. Obtain another PSA test, if again elevated, then...
5. Obtain a DCE-MRI or color Doppler ultrasound, then...
6. Avoid a blind biopsy and, if needed get a targeted biopsy via color Doppler ultrasound or DCR-MRI-guided biopsy, then...
7. If biopsy reveals cancer, consider getting a second pathology analysis from a different center or institution, or consider genetic testing, then...
8. If the biopsy is negative but PSA keeps rising, consider genetic testing...
9. Join a support group, do your research and search the Internet, then...
10. Collect your data, assess it with your doctor, ask questions, then...
11. If necessary, consider getting a second opinion, then...
12. Decide on treatment.

2011-2020: THE RENAISSANCE DECADE OF TREATING PROSTATE CANCER

Imagine, when the diagnostic technologies and new therapies like these become widely used, almost everything about prostate cancer care will change. Soon, patients and their doctors will wonder why there ever was a debate about the DCE-MRI and MRI-guided biopsy, about genetic testing and alpharadin, and how did we ever get along without them. These next ten years are going to be the renaissance decade of prostate cancer care, a time of amazing departure from the past in the diagnosis and treatment of this very common and all-too-often lethal cancer in men.

It is already underway. I had lunch with Charles Mason the other day. We have been friends for nearly forty years. In April 2011, his PSA rose to 4.5 ng/ml. This is only slightly above normal, but it was double the previous PSA level a year before, which was worrisome. His urologist recommended a biopsy, which did not detect cancer. However, the day after the biopsy, Charlie developed chills and fever. He was already taking an antibiotic for the biopsy, but it obviously had not prevented infection from the biopsy. His doctor switched antibiotics, yet Charles worsened. Two days later, he was in the hospital receiving intravenous antibiotics. The first one didn't work, the second caused a severe rash, and meanwhile Charles' condition deteriorated. He almost died.

Finally a third antibiotic brought the infection under control. It was a close call for Charles, because the last antibiotic began causing kidney failure. If the drug hadn't controlled the infection quickly, it would have had to be discontinued and at this point there were few other treatment choices.

When Charles and I had lunch recently, I asked about his latest PSA level. "I am putting it off," he admitted. "I know I shouldn't, but I am worried it will come back elevated and I will have to undergo another biopsy. I dread that."

Charles knew I had prostate cancer but didn't know the details of my journey. I gave him the short version and then suggested he get a prostate DCE-MRI.

He took a minute to think this over, then he said, "You know, that's not a bad idea. If the PSA remains elevated, I will need a biopsy again, and a prostate DCE-MRI might show us where to look. Even if the PSA is normal, I will still worry that we might be missing something." He smiled. "I've had MRIs for my shoulder and lower back. Why not get one for the prostate and see what's really going on?"

I added, "And if the DCE-MRI shows no cancer, then you can wait on the biopsy without worry. If the MRI shows suspicious areas, you can get a guided biopsy. With a guided biopsy, they will only need a few cores from the lesion. With a blind biopsy, they will take 12 or 14 cores. So your risk of injury and infection would be much less with a guided biopsy. The fewer biopsy cores, the better, especially with you, but really with all men."

"That makes a lot of sense," Charles said. "It's nice to know I have options."

Charles did get a DCE-MRI, which showed a small abnormality, possibly cancer, in a safe area. Charles' PSA had dropped, so Charles and his urologist agreed to monitor his PSA levels and repeat the DCE-MRI before doing another biopsy. In essence, even though cancer has never been diagnosed, Charles is doing active surveillance.

TO THE WOMEN WHO ARE READING THIS BOOK

Thank you. You must care very much about your husband, boyfriend, father, son, brother or other men in your life. This is so important, because one of every six men you know or have ever known will develop prostate cancer.

Women read health books more often than men. Some men with prostate cancer are avid readers, but many men just want to "deal with it," meaning action, meaning surgery or radiation. Some men need these aggressive therapies, but many more do not. Women reading this book can help steer their men to doctors who are informed about the new tests and treatments.

I greatly admire the work women have done during the past twenty years in raising awareness about breast cancer. Pink ribbons and breast cancer walks and fundraisers have done much to advance our knowledge about screening, testing and treatment. Men have taken a lesson and prostate cancer support groups are growing, but we are far behind the ladies. I tip my hat.

In the great majority of cases of prostate cancer, there is time to obtain all of the useful diagnostic tests. With these, treatment decisions become easier, and for many men, safer. If some women have to push their men to follow the approach I have spelled out in *Prostate Cancer Breakthroughs*, you have provided your men a great service.

KNOWLEDGE IS POWER

The goal of this book has been to alert you to the breakthrough tests and treatments available today for men with prostate cancer. Each test you obtain can provide additional information that can make your treatment decision easier and more precise. In my case and in other men I have mentioned here, the DCE-MRI or color Doppler ultrasound changed everything. Knowing specifically the size, type, location, and absence of spread of my prostate cancer allowed me to consider an option that had been off the table, active surveillance. I have been following this method for 22 months and feel comfortable with it. At least, as comfortable as a man can feel who has been diagnosed with prostate cancer.

More than half of the men diagnosed with prostate cancer today are candidates for active surveillance, yet most of them undergo prostatectomy or radiation despite the risk of long-term harm to their quality of life. In addition, prostatectomy and radiation treatment are not cures for 20-25% of men who undergo them. Yes, some men do require a prostatectomy or radiation, but others who undergo these treatments really don't need them. Current methods do not provide most men with enough information to make a truly informed decision. Many men are not even told about the focal therapies that would make sense for them. Making a diagnosis based solely on PSA levels and a blind biopsy, as most doctors do today, are simply not enough. The new tests, which can give you a picture of what you have and what you need to do, can change that.

Consider that 1,200,000 men in the U.S. undergo a prostate biopsy each year, yet only half of them need it.[4] Prostate biopsies are usually safe, but as you saw in Richard's case, prostate biopsies do have serious risks and in nearly one in 1,000 men are fatal. Why rush into a biopsy, which is a surgical procedure, before finding out via a prostate MRI or color Doppler ultrasound if you actually need one?

This is why I encourage you to obtain *all the tests you can, and all the second opinions you need* to be fully informed about what you have and what you need to do. *You have cancer.* If ever there was time for you to be assertive and ask questions about tests and treatments, it is now.

ACKNOWLEDGMENTS

I want to express my deep appreciation to the Informed Prostate Cancer Support Group. The willingness of its members to reach out and educate men like me who are newly diagnosed prostate cancer is both generous and invaluable. Their efforts changed the course of my medical care for the better. Groups like IPCSG are helpful not only for supporting men with this terrible and sometimes deadly cancer, but also in spreading the word about vital new tests and treatments, ideas that men with prostate cancer can take to their doctors, thereby facilitating much needed change in the medical approach to prostate cancer care today. For readers of this book, the IPCSG website (ipcsg.org) is an excellent source of information, particularly the monthly lectures and discussions, available on DVD, with top experts in all of the fields of medicine that are involved in the treatment of prostate cancer.

My sincere thanks also to the small group of fellows who meet every week over Chinese food to discuss our individual challenges as well as new ideas and reports about prostate cancer.

I also want to thank my publication team of Beth and Ezra Barany of Barany Consulting, and my reliable proofreaders, Karen Lockwood and Barbara Isrow-Cohen. Thank you for your guidance, support and encouragement in my new adventure as both writer and publisher. It has been an ongoing learning experience and a thrill.

REFERENCES

Introduction: A Better Approach to Prostate Cancer

1. Fang F, Fall K, Mittleman MA, et al. Suicide and cardiovascular death after a cancer diagnosis. New England Journal of Medicine Apr 5, 2012;366:1310-18.
2. Blum RH, Scholz M. Invasion of the Prostate Snatchers: An essential guide to managing prostate cancer for patients and their families. 2011, Other Press, New York, NY.

Section 1: The Key: A More Accurate Diagnostic Approach

Step 1: Why You Must Get an Annual PSA Test

1. United States Preventive Services Task Force. Screening for Prostate Cancer: Current Recommendation. May 2012: http://www.usp reventiveservicestaskforce.org/prostatecancerscreening.htm
2. Carter HB, Albertsen PC, Barry MJ, et al. Early detection of prostate cancer: AUA Guideline. American Urological Association, May 2013: www.auanet.org.
3. Jacobs BL, Zhang Y, Schroeck FR, et al. Use of advanced treatment technologies among men at low risk of dying from prostate cancer. JAMA 2013, Jun 26;309(24):2587 95.
4. Schröder FH, Hugosson J, Roobol MJ, et al. Prostate cancer mortality at 11 years of follow up. N Engl J Med. 2012 Mar 15;366(11):981 90.
5. Loeb S, Vonesh EF, Metter EJ, et al. What is the true number needed to screen and treat to save a life with prostate specific antigen testing? Journal of Clinical Oncology 2011, Feb 1;29(4):464 7.
6. Blum RH, Scholz M. Invasion of the Prostate Snatchers: An essential guide to managing prostate cancer for patients and their families. 2011, Other Press, New York, NY.

Step 2: Blind Biopsy, Targeted Biopsy, or No Biopsy?

1. Nam RK, Saskin R, Lee Y, et al. Increasing hospital admission rates for urological complications after transrectal ultrasound guided prostate biopsy. J Urol. 2013 Jan;189(1 Suppl):S12-7; discussion S17-8.

2. The impact of repeat biopsies on infectious complications in men with prostate cancer on active surveillance: a prospective study. Abstract 1244. New Prostate Cancer Infolink, May 1, 2013: http://prostatecancerinfolink.net/2013/05/01/risks-associated-with-serial-biopsies-for-men-on-active-surveillance-protocols/#comment-42083

3. Blum RH, Scholz M. Invasion of the Prostate Snatchers: An essential guide to managing prostate cancer for patients and their families. 2011, Other Press, New York, NY.

4. Marks L, Young S, Natarajan S. MRI-ultrasound fusion for guidance of targeted prostate biopsy. Current Opinion-Urology 2013, Jan;23(1):43-50.

Step 5: The New, Contrast-Enhanced, Prostate MRI (DCE-MRI)

1. Chodak G. Winning the battle against prostate cancer. 2011, Demos Medical Publishing, New York, NY.

2. Cohen JS. Over Dose: The Case Against The Drug Companies. Prescription Drugs, Side Effects, and Your Health. Tarcher-Putnam New York: October 2001.

3. Lazarou J, Pomeranz BH, Corey PN. Incidence of adverse drug reactions in hospitalized patients: a meta analysis of prospective studies. JAMA 1998;279(15):1200 5.

4. Sackett DL, Rosenberg WM, Gray JA, et al. Evidence-Based Medicine: What it is and what it isn't. Centre for Evidence-Based Medicine: www.ncbi.nlm.nih.gov/pmc/articles/PMC2349778, May 14, 2004.

5. Sackett DL, Straus SE, Richardson WS, et al. Evidence-Based Medicine: How to Practice and Teach EBM. 2000, Churchill Livingstone: Edinburgh.

6. Than M, Bidwell S, Davison C, et al. Evidence based emergency medicine at the 'coal face.' Emergency Medicine Australasia 2005;17(4):330 40.

7. Miller FG, Rosenstein DL. The therapeutic orientation to clinical trials. New England Journal of Medicine 2003;384:1383-1386.

8. Guyatt G, Rennie D. Users' Guide to the Medical Literature: a Manual for Evidence-Based Clinical Practice. 2002, American Medical Association: Chicago.
9. Puech P, Potiron E, Lemaitre L, et al. Dynamic Contrast enhanced Magnetic Resonance Imaging Evaluation of Intraprostatic Prostate Cancer: Correlation with Radical Prostatectomy Specimens. Urology 2009;74:1094-1100.
10. Scardino PT, Kellman J. Dr. Peter Scardino's Prostate Book. 2010, Avery Books: New York, NY.
11. Beck M. The Man, the Gland, the Dilemmas. Wall Street Journal, March 31, 2009.
12. Ibid.

Step 6: The Color Doppler Ultrasound

1. Dr. Duke Bahn on color Doppler ultrasound. Ask Dr. Myers, Oct. 10, 2013: https://askdrmyers.wordpress.com/2013/10/10/dr-duke-bahn-on-color-doppler-ultrasound.
1A. Sen J, Choudhary L, Marwah S, et al. Role of color Doppler imaging in detecting prostate cancer. Asian Journal of Surgery 2008;31(1):16-19.
2. Navratil F. Letter, Wall Street Journal, April 7, 2010: prostablog.wordpress.com/older-stuff/articles/wall-st-journal-prostate-articles\. Accessed June 21, 2012.

Step 7: Genetic Diagnostic Tests that Are Available Now

1. Pollack A. New prostate cancer tests could reduce false alarms. New York Times Mar. 26, 2013: nytimes.com/2013/03/27/business/new-prostate-cancer-tests-may-supplement-psa-testing.html?pagewanted=all&_r=0.
2. Foster DJ. New biomarker tests for prostate cancer. PCRI (Prostate Cancer Research Institute) newsletter, Aug. 2013; 16(3): http://prostate-cancer.org/wp-content/uploads/insights/august 2013/Insights_August2013_%20New_Biomarker_Test.pdf

Step 8: The New, Carbon-11 PET/CT Scans for Metastatic Prostate Cancer

1. National Institutes of Health (NIH). C-11 Choline PET-CT Scan in Finding Metastases in Patients with Newly Diagnosed High-Risk Prostate Cancer. http://clinicaltrials.gov/show/NCT00804245

2. Chang AJ, Seo Y, Behr S, Roach M. The Utility of C-11 Choline PET/CT for Prostate Cancer: Improving Detection of Locoregional and Metastatic Disease. http://gucasym.asco.org/utility-c-11-choline-petct-prostate-cancer-improving-detection-locoregional-and-metastatic-disease

Section Two: A Broader Range of Treatment Options for Men with Prostate Cancer

A. Aggressive Therapies

Option 1: Prostatectomy

1. Sinnott M, Falzarano SM, Hernandez AV, et al. Discrepancy in prostate cancer localization between biopsy and prostatectomy specimens in patients with unilateral positive biopsy: implications for focal therapy. Prostate 2012, Aug. 1;72(11):1175-86.
2. Eifler JB, Humphreys EB, Agro M, et al. Causes of death after radical prostatectomy at a large tertiary center. Journal of Urology, Sept. 2012;188(3):798-802.
3. Menon M, Bhandari M, Gupta N et al. Biochemical recurrence following robot-persisted radical prostatectomy. European Urology 2010;58:838-846.
4. Eastham J, Scardino PT, Kattan MW. Predicting an optimal outcome after radical prostatectomy: the trifecta nomogram. Journal of Urology, June 2008;179:2207-10.

Option 2-5: Radiation Therapies - IMRT, SBRT (CyberKnife), Proton, Brachytherapy

1. Katz AJ, Santoro M, Diblasio F, Ashley R. Stereotactic body radiotherapy for localized prostate cancer: disease control and quality of life at 6 years. Radiation Oncology, 2013 May 13;8(1):118.
1A. Allen AM, Pawlicki T, Dong L, et al. An evidence based review of proton beam therapy: the report of ASTRO's emerging technology committee. Radiotherapy and Oncology, Apr 2012;103(1):8-11.
1B. Terhune C. Blue Shield of California to curb coverage of pricey cancer therapy. Los Angeles Times, 2013, Aug. 29: .latimes.com/business/la-fi-hospital-proton-beam-20130829,0,1343046.story.

2. Zelefsky MJ, Pei X, Teslova T, et al. Secondary cancers after intensity-modulated radiotherapy, brachytherapy and radical prostatectomy for the treatment of prostate cancer. BJU International 2012; Aug. 13:1464-1410.

3. Vora SA, Wong WW, Schild SE, et al. Analysis of biochemical control and prognostic factors in patients treated with either low-dose three-dimensional conformal radiation therapy or doctors IMRT for localized prostate cancer. International Journal of Radiation Oncology, Biology, Physics, July 15, 2007;68(4):1053-58.

4. Alicikus ZA, Yamada Y, Zhang Z, et al. Ten-year outcomes of high-dose, intensity-modulated radiotherapy [IMRT] for localized prostate cancer. Cancer 2011, Apr. 1;117(7):1429-37.

5. Pradat PF, Poisson M, Delattre JY, et al. Radiation induced neuropathies: experimental and clinical data. Revue Neurology 1994 Oct;150(10):664 77.

6. Chen AM, Hall WH, Li J, et al. Brachial Plexus Associated Neuropathy After High Dose Radiation Therapy for Head and Neck Cancer. International Journal of Radiation and Oncology, Biology and Physics 2012, Mar 21: Epub.

7. Gikas PD, Hanna SA, Aston W, et al. Post radiation sciatic neuropathy: a case report and review of the literature. World Journal of Surgery and Oncology, Dec 2008;11(6):130.

8. Johansson S, Svensson H, Denekamp J. International Journal of Radiation and Oncology, Biology and Physics, Apr 2002;52(5):1207 19.

9. Rubin DI, Schomberg PJ, Shepherd RF, Panneton JM. Arteritis and brachial plexus neuropathy as delayed complications of radiation therapy. Mayo Clinic Proceedings, Aug 2001;76(8):849 52.

10. Lalu T, Mercier B, Birouk N, et al. Pure motor neuropathy after radiation therapy: 6 cases. Revue Neurology (Paris), Jan 1998;154(1):40 4.

11. Royal College Radiologists. Management of radiation induced brachial plexus neuropathy. Oncology (Williston Park), May 1996;10(5):685, 689.

12. Stoll BA, Andrews JT. Radiation induced Peripheral Neuropathy. British Medical Journal, Apr 2, 1966;1(5491):834 7.

B. Focal Therapies

1. Sperling D. Focal laser ablation of prostate tumors. Choices, the PAACTUSA newsletter, Dec. 2012:14-17, paactusa.org.
2. Beck M. The Man, the Gland, the Dilemmas. Wall Street Journal, March 31, 2009.

Option 6: Cryotherapy

1. Dr. Duke Bahn on color Doppler ultrasound. Ask Dr. Myers, Oct. 10, 2013: https://askdrmyers.wordpress.com/2013/10/10/dr-duke-bahn-on-color-doppler-ultrasound.
1A. Bahn DK, Silverman P, Lee F, et al. Focal process cryoablation initial results show cancer controls and potency preservation. Journal of Endourology 2006;20(9):688-92.

Option: 7: Focal Laser Ablation (FLA)

1. Sperling D. Focal laser ablation of prostate tumors. Choices, the PAACTUSA Newsletter, Dec. 2012:14-17, paactusa.org.
2. Springen K. New hope for men with prostate cancer. Chicago Mag.com, July 2011: http://www.chicagomag.com/Chicago-Magazine/July-2011/New-Hope-For-Men-With-Prostate-Cancer.
3. Molly Dannenmaier. Nonsurgical prostate cancer treatment: a first of kind in Texas. Galveston County Daily News, May 14, 2013: http://www.utmb.edu/newsroom/article8543.aspx.

Option 8: High Intensity Focused Ultrasound (HIFU)

1. Sung HH, Jeong BC, Seo SI, et al. Seven years experience with high-intensity focused ultrasound for prostate cancer: advantages and limitations. Prostate 2012, Sep 15;72(13):1399-1406.
2. Zini C, Hipp E, Thomas S, et al. Ultrasound- and MR-guided focused ultrasound surgery for prostate cancer. World Journal of Radiology 2012, June 28;4(6):247-252.
3. Ahmed HU, Freeman A, Kirkham A, et al. Focal therapy for localized prostate cancer: a phase I/II trial. Journal of Urology 2011;185(4):1246-55.

C. Non-invasive Therapies

Option 9: Medication Therapy

1. Blum RH, Scholz M. Invasion of the Prostate Snatchers: An essential guide to managing prostate cancer for patients and their families. 2011, Other Press, New York, NY.
2. Scholz M, Lam R, Strum S, et al. Primary intermittent androgen deprivation as initial therapy for men with newly diagnosed prostate cancer. Clinical Genitourinary Cancer 2011, Dec;9(2):89-94.

Option 10: Active Surveillance: More Than Watching and Waiting

1. Parker-Pope T. Choosing watchful waiting for prostate cancer. New York Times, July 23, 2012.
2. Ibid.
2A. Marks L. Ultrasound-MRI Fusion for Targeted Diagnosis of Prostate Cancer: Use of Artemis Device to Evaluate Organ-Confined Lesions. http://casit.ucla.edu/body.cfm?id=222. Accessed 8-22-13.
3. Wilt TJ, Brawer MK, Jones KM, et al. Radical prostatectomy vs. observation for localized prostate cancer. New England Journal of Medicine, July 19, 2012; 367(3):203-2012.
4. Parker-Pope T. Questioning Surgery for Early Prostate Cancer. Wall Street Journal, July 18, 2012.
5. 1. Dr. Duke Bahn on color Doppler ultrasound. Ask Dr. Myers, Oct. 10, 2013: https://askdrmyers.wordpress.com/2013/10/10/dr-duke-bahn-on-color-doppler-ultrasound.
6. National Institutes of Health. The role of active surveillance in the management of men with localized prostate cancer. NIH Consensus and State-of-the-Science Statements, Dec. 7, 2011, 28(1):6.

Option 11: Alpharadin for Bone Metastases

1. U.S. Food and Drug Administration. FDA approves new drug for advanced prostate cancer. May 15, 2013:www.fda.gov.
2. Bayer Pharmaceuticals. A Phase 3 study of radium-223 dichloride in patients with symptomatic hormone refractory prostate cancer with skeletal metastases (ALSYMPCA). Identifier NCT00699751. ClinicalTrials.gov, a Service of the U.S. National Institutes of Health.
3. Parker C, Nilsson S, Heinrich D, et al. Alpha emitter radium-223 and survival in metastatic prostate cancer. New England Journal Medincine 2013, Jul 18;369(3):213-23.

Option 12: Too Good to be True? Proscar (Finasteride) to Prevent Prostate Cancer

1. Marchione M. Drug cuts prostate cancer risk, study finds. Associated Press, San Diego Union-Tribune, 2013, Aug. 15:A13.
1A. Thompson IM, Goodman PJ, Tangen CM, et al. Long-Term survival of participants in the prostate cancer prevention trial. New England Journal of Medicine, Aug. 15, 2013;369:603-610.
2. Thompson IM, Goodman PJ, Tangen CM, et al. The influence of finasteride on the development of prostate cancer. New England Journal of Medicine July 17, 2003349:215-224.
3. Scardino PT. The prevention of prostate cancer—the dilemma continues. New England Journal of Medicine, July 17, 2003;349:297-299.
4. Physicians' Desk Reference, 67th Edition. Montvale, NJ: PDR Network, 2013.
5. Reinberg S. Sexual side effects from Propecia, Avodart may be irreversible. USA Today, Mar. 13, 2011: http://usatoday30.usatoday.com/news/health/medical/health/medical/menshealth/story/2011/03/Sexual-side-effects-from-Propecia-Avodart-may-be-irreversible/44787684/1
6. Traish AM, Hassani J, Guay AT, Zitzmann M, Hansen ML. Adverse side effects of 5α-reductase inhibitors therapy: persistent diminished libido and erectile dysfunction and depression in a subset of patients. Journal of Sexual Medicine, Mar. 2011;8(3):872-84.

7. NPR News. Evidence supports pill to prevent some prostate cancers. Aug. 14, 2013: http://www.npr.org/blogs/health/2013/08/14/21 2046489/evidence-supports-pill-to-prevent-some-prostate-cancers

Section 3: Weighing the Evidence and Making a Decision

Step 9: What Does Your Data Say?

1. Blum RH, Scholz M. Invasion of the Prostate Snatchers: An essential guide to managing prostate cancer for patients and their families. 2011, Other Press, New York, NY.
2. Katz AE. The definitive guide to prostate cancer. 2011, Rodale Press: New York, NY.
3. Scardino PT, Kellman J. Dr. Peter Scardino's Prostate Book. 2010, Avery Books: New York, NY.
4. Wilt TJ, Brawer MK, Jones KM, et al. Radical prostatectomy vs. observation for localized prostate cancer. New England Journal of Medicine, July 19, 2012; 367(3):203-2012.
5. Pollack A. New prostate cancer tests could reduce false alarms. New York Times Mar. 26, 2013: nytimes.com/2013/03/27/business/new -prostate-cancer-tests-may-supplement-psa- testing.html?pagewanted=all&_r=0.
6. Cohen, JS. Peripheral Neuropathy with Fluoroquinolone Antibiotics. Annals of Pharmacotherapy, Dec. 2001;35(12):1540-47.

PEER- REVIEWED MEDICAL JOURNAL PUBLICATIONS BY JAY S. COHEN, M.D.

You can see additional articles by Dr. Cohen at his websites:
- ProstateCancerBreakthroughs.com
- MedicationSense.com
- JayCohenMD.com

Cohen JS. Peripheral Neuropathy with Fluoroquinolone Antibiotics (Cipro, Levaquin, Avelox). *Annals of Pharmacotherapy*, Dec. 2001;35(12):1540-47.

Cohen JS. Statin therapy after stroke or transient ischemic attack. *New England Journal of Medicine* 2006;355(22):2368.

Cohen JS. Risks of troglitazone (Rezulin) apparent before approval in USA. Diabetologia 2006;49(6):1454-5.

Cohen JS. How celecoxib (Celebrex) could be safer; how valdecoxib (Bextra) might have been. Annals of Pharmacotherapy, Sept. 2005;39:1542-1545.

Cohen JS. Should rosuvastatin (Crestor) be withdrawn from the market [letter]? Lancet, Oct. 2004;364(9445):1579.

Cohen JS. Antidepressants: An avoidable and solvable controversy. *Annals of Pharmacotherapy*, Oct. 2004;38(10):1743-1746.

Cohen JS. Magnesium and erythromelalgia: a clinically important vasoactive mineral and a rare disorder. *Italian Journal of Pediatrics* 2004;30:69-72.

Cohen JS. Statins and low density lipoprotein cholesterol levels [letter]. *American Journal of Medicine*, July 2003;115(1):74 75

Cohen JS. Do Standard Doses of Frequently Prescribed Drugs Cause Preventable Adverse Effects in Women? *JAMWA (The Journal of the American Medical Women's Association)* 2002;57:105-110.

Cohen JS. Why Aren't Lower, Effective, OTC Doses Available Earlier by Prescription? *Annals of Pharmacotherapy*, Jan. 2003;37(1):136-142.

Cohen JS. Tablet Splitting: Imperfect Perhaps, but Better Than Excessive Dosing. *Journal of the American Pharmacy Association*, Mar. 2002;42(2):160-162.

Cohen JS. High-Dose, Oral Magnesium in the Treatment of Chronic, Intractable Erythromelalgia. *Annals of Pharmacotherapy*, Feb. 2002;36:255-60.

Cohen JS. Pharmaceutical manufacturer sponsorship and drug information [letter]. *Archives of Internal Medicine*, Nov. 26, 2001;161:2625-2626.

Cohen JS. Clinical and Ethical Concerns about Switching Patient Treatment to "Therapeutically Interchangeable" Medications [letter]. *Archives of Internal Medicine*, Sept. 24, 2001;161:2153-54.

Cohen JS. Dose Discrepancies between the Physicians' Desk Reference and the Medical Literature, and Their Possible Role in the High Incidence of Dose-Related Adverse Drug Events. *Archives of Internal Medicine*, April 9, 2001:161:957-64.

Cohen JS. Adverse drug effects, compliance, and the initial doses of antihypertensive drugs recommended by the Joint National Committee vs. the Physicians' Desk Reference. *Archives of Internal Medicine*, March 26, 2001;161:880-85.

Cohen JS. Comparison of FDA Reports of Patient Deaths Associated with Sildenafil (Viagra) and with Injectable Alprostadil (Caverject). *Annals of Pharmacotherapy*, March 2001;35:285-88.

Cohen JS. Is the Product Information on Sildenafil (Viagra) Adequate to Facilitate Optimal Therapeutics and to Minimize Adverse Events? *Annals of Pharmacotherapy*, March 2001;35:337-42.

Cohen JS. Erythromelalgia: New Theories and New Therapies. *Journal of the American Academy of Dermatology*, Nov. 2000;43:841-7.

Cohen JS. Should Patients Be Given a Low Test Dose of sildenafil (Viagra) Initially? *Drug Safety* July 2000;23:1-10.

Cohen JS. Adverse Drug Reactions: Effective Low-Dose Therapies for Older Patients. *Geriatrics* Feb. 2000;55(2):54-64.

Cohen JS. Viagra and Nonnitrate Antihypertensive Medications (letter). *JAMA*, Jan 12, 2000;283(2):201 2.

Cohen JS. The One-Size Dose Does Not Fit All: Look beyond the guidelines of drug manufacturers. *Newsweek*, Dec. 6, 1999:92.

Cohen JS. Preventing Adverse Drug Reactions Before They Occur. Expert Pharmacology Column. *Medscap*e (www.Medscape.com), Dec 1999.

Cohen JS. Ways To Minimize Adverse Drug Reactions: Individualized Doses and Common Sense Are Key. *Postgraduate Medicine* 1999;106:163-72.

Cohen JS., Insel PA. The Physicians' Desk Reference. Problems and possible improvements. *Archives of Internal Medicine* 1996;156(13):1375 80.

Cohen JS. Dosage titration issues [letter]. *Journal of Clinical Psychiatry*, January 1996.

Cohen JS. Provide fluoxetine (Prozac) information vital to clinicians [letter]. *Journal of Clinical Psychiatry*, Dec 1995.

Cohen JS. Is alprazolam (Xanax) the best treatment for panic attacks [letter]. *Journal of Clinical Psychiatry*, August 1988.

ABOUT THE AUTHOR

Jay Cohen M.D. is a nationally respected expert on prescription medications and side effects, a driving force for the implementation of better methods to reduce the high rate of medication-related deaths (150,000) and hospitalizations (2,000,000) annually in America. He is also an expert on natural remedies.

Dr. Cohen earned his medical degree at Temple University, Philadelphia, in 1971. After completing his internship, he practiced general medicine and subsequently conducted ground-breaking research at UCLA in 1973 on acupuncture and pain. In 1974, he undertook a residency in psychiatry and psychopharmacology at the University of California, San Diego, where today he is an Adjunct (voluntary) Associate Professor of Psychiatry. He is also the Chairman of the Medical Advisory Committee of The Erythromelalgia Association, as well as a Fellow of the American College of Nutrition.

Dr. Cohen's favorite subject in medical school was pharmacology and it remains so. Since then, Dr. Cohen has performed independent research in pharmacology, specifically on the causes of medication side effects. The emphasis of his work has been on prevention. Dr. Cohen's identification of a substantial proportion of the population that is medication-sensitive has been groundbreaking. Since 1988, he has published his findings in 8 books and leading medical journals, as well as articles in consumer publications such as *Newsweek, Bottom Line Health*, and *Life Extension Magazine*. Dr. Cohen's work has been featured in the *New York Times, Washington Post, Consumer Reports, Wall Street Journal, Modern Maturity, Women's Day*, and virtually every major magazine and newspaper in America. His book, *Over Dose: The Case Against The Drug Companies* (Tarcher/Putnam, Nov. 2001), received unanimously excellent reviews from Publishers Weekly, Library Journal and the *Journal of the American Medical Association*.

Dr. Cohen has been featured on more than 200 radio programs across America including the "People's Pharmacy" and National Public Radio. He has spoken at conferences of patients, doctors, drug industry executives, and attorneys. In October 2001, during the anthrax scare, his medical journal article on severe reactions to Cipro, Levaquin, and other fluoroquinolone antibiotics triggered a national debate on the best treatment for anthrax and prompted the U.S. Centers for Disease Control to withdraw its recommendation for the use of these antibiotics in anthrax exposure cases. In November 2002, Dr. Cohen was the keynote speaker at the Annual Science Day of the U.S. Food and Drug Administration's Clinical Pharmacology Division. He has debated top FDA officials on drug safety at conferences including the American Society for Clinical Pharmacology and Therapeutics and the Drug Information Association. You can see more about his work in these areas at his website MedicationSense.com, as well as his work in anxiety and depressive disorders, and people who are sensitive to medications, at JayCohenMD.com.

Dr. Cohen conducts his research, writing and office practice in Del Mar, CA. Dr. Cohen wrote *Prostate Cancer Breakthroughs* after being diagnosed with the disease in December 2011. Originally released in March 2013, the book quickly became a best-seller and remains #1 at Amazon.com today (11-19-13) among books on prostate cancer.

Because of the many advances in prostate cancer care during 2013, Dr. Cohen rewrote the book including a new section on the importance of PSA testing (despite the de-emphasis of PSA testing by federal panels and the medical establishment). He also increased the number of medical centers, from 8 to 24, offering DCE-MRI testing for prostate cancer. In addition, Dr. Cohen added new sections on genetic testing, Carbon-11 PET/CT testing for prostate cancer metastases, medication therapy for prostate cancer, alpharadin therapy for metastatic prostate cancer, and CyberKnife radiation therapy. Overall, 52 pages of new information were added to the original 2013 edition of the book.

Today, *Prostate Cancer Breakthroughs 2014* remains the most comprehensive, up-to-date, step-by-step guide for diagnosing and treating prostate cancer effectively.

MORE READERS' REVIEWS OF PROSTATE CANCER BREAKTHROUGHS

5/5 Stars: "If you or a man you know has prostate cancer, this book is a 'must read.' Presented without bias by a medical professional who is not a prostate cancer doctor, but instead, a patient. His objectivity is refreshing among all the other books on this subject. He ends with: You have cancer. If there was ever a time to ask questions and demand answers... It is now!" *Ray M., Plano, TX, Aug. 27, 2013*

5/5 Stars: "Dr. Cohen is top notch! Sixteen years ago I had a prostatectomy. It was unnecessary. But, I had no books like that from Jay. He is open and courageous. He is helpful. Tells it like it is. I am glad to have the book and thankful to Dr. Cohen." *John L., May 22, 2013.*

5/5 Stars: "Excellent and the latest on the new approaches. I thoroughly enjoyed this book and it helped me a lot with my plight with prostate cancer. The section about MRI-guided laser ablation was especially helpful." *Clark, August 22, 2013.*

5/5 Stars: "This is precisely the type of book I would want to get my hands on had I just been diagnosed with prostate cancer. It is so important that you and I as patients take the lead in researching the options and making informed treatment choices. Dr. Cohen's book provides a step-by-step guide that is easy to follow and understand." *C.T., May 27, 2013.*

5/5 Stars: "A must-read for all men over the age of 40! I recently read Dr. Jay Cohen's book about Prostate Cancer, and was very impressed by the clear presentation of the dilemma that many men will face during their lifetime. This book is extremely important for men to read before they plan a diagnostic procedure, since diagnosis is the single most important aspect of prostate cancer. As Dr. Cohen explains, in recent times, extremely accurate testing procedures and equipment have been developed. The book is a real treasure, a bargain, and could save your life!" *M.B., April 23, 2013.*

5/5 Stars: "Having been written by an MD without any oncology training gives this book great credibility. The author set out to get an education before he made decisions about his treatment. With all respect to surgeons, their desire to cut immediately is often offered as the only solution. As Dr. Cohen found out and explains clearly the need to explore other treatment options is necessary before making life changing treatment decisions." *Bill B., Englewood, Fl, July 12, 2013*

5/5 Stars: "A MUST FOR EVERY ADULT MAN. This is an unbelievably beautiful, timely, and candid book. The author is an MD with outstanding credentials. If you read his 2001 book OVER DOSE: THE CASE AGAINST THE DRUG COMPANIES, you'll see he doesn't pull his punches. A shining gem in this book is Cohen's argument on page 79, using a study conducted at the Cleveland Clinic and published in 2012, that of 179 men who underwent radical prostatectomy (removal of the prostate and more) between 2004 and 2008, about 71% had not needed the surgery. ... Read this nice, concise book and you will find out all there is to know about new tests, new treatments, and better options in the treatment of prostate cancer. Afterwards, chances are you will know more than most urologists and radiologists. What more can you ask for the price of a couple of beers at the ballpark?" *Flying Samaritan, April 17, 2013.*

5/5 Stars: "As a practicing clinician, one of the most frustrating aspects of men's health has been incorrect diagnosis and unnecessary treatment based on PSA levels. Dr. Cohen, a long time advocate for honest medicine and champion of patient advocacy who established his mark with his courageous book OVER DOSE, has written a guide for men and their doctors on how to best approach evaluation of prostate cancer. Every man and every doctor needs to take a serious look at this little book." *J. E. Williams, OMD, April 22, 2013.*

5/5 Stars: "I have strongly recommended this book to my medical colleagues, patients, family, and friends who are dealing with concerns about prostate cancer. Dr. Cohen clearly describes the process of thoughtful evaluation with the latest technologies. And he correctly cautions the reader against blindly rushing in for procedures that may not be necessary and, perhaps, cause harm. This book is well researched, clearly written, and contains actionable information. It's a must read." *Dan G. M.D., July 24, 2013.*

5/5 Stars: "BEST MEDICAL ADVICE OF MY LIFE—COULD NOT PUT THIS BOOK DOWN! After reading Dr. Cohen's incredible book, the anxiety I have felt concerning my prostate for over 15 years has finally subsided. Fifteen years ago I was told that I had BPH—who doesn't—LOL! Several PSA tests and a few years later, I was told to have a prostate biopsy, which I declined in favor of a "second opinion" from a renowned "expert urologist". He told me that aside from BPH, my prostate seemed perfectly normal. He then referred me to one of his "protégées." My PSA levels continued to fluctuate, and I experienced a severe case of prostatitis. I continued my follow up visits with the docs on that team, none of whom would appropriately "listen" or "explain" their "recommendations" which included heavy doses of antibiotics and a biopsy, all of which I declined. I subsequently decided to find another urologist, and found an excellent one. Although my symptoms persisted, I have been pursuing a course of "active surveillance" (as Dr. Cohen describes as a viable option in this book). Before reading Dr. Cohen's book, I had been searching for answers and information regarding my condition. I now feel that I had made the appropriate decisions about myself. This book has detailed, described, and discussed every question and concern I have had but could neither articulate nor find answers for. What a relief! Finally, I feel that I am now in control of my options. I will continue to pursue a prudent course of active surveillance, and before I undergo any invasive tests, I will DEMAND the options recommended by Dr. Cohen. My advice to anyone who has any issues or questions about their prostate is to READ THIS BOOK! Don't make any decisions or undergo any procedures until you have discussed the options and recommendations presented by Cohen with your urologist." *FA ONE, April 17, 2013.*

5/5 Stars: "A must-read for all men and the women who love them. I got this book for background information for an article I was writing on prostate health for a national publication. I meant just to skim through it, but I couldn't put it down—I read it cover to cover! A mere 100 pages [now larger], Dr. Cohen's book is a clear, concise, step-by-step guide for negotiating the often murky maze of medical testing and treatment for prostate cancer, complete with information about where to receive cutting edge care. The explanations of various tests and treatments are easy to understand and also well balanced—with pros and cons of each option explained. I only wish this book was available a year ago, when a close friend had prostate cancer and needed this kind of information." *Medwriter, April 17, 2013.*

5/5 Stars: "READ THIS BOOK! A must read for any man who has a PSA test (all men should at any age), and for men just diagnosed with prostate cancer. Dr. Jay Cohen's Prostate Cancer Breakthroughs is current, concise, and understandable. The information is cutting edge with new, game-changing diagnostic tests and treatment possibilities that will help many men avoid radical surgery or radiation." *L. Romane, M.D., May 28, 2013.*

5/5 Stars: "Very good and credible information from a doctor who knows his business. Would highly recommend it for everyone's medical knowledge in this area." *boomersooner, Plano, Tx, July 25, 2013.*

4/5 Stars: "A thought provoking book for anyone who is contemplating treatment for prostate cancer. I would recommend this to all men....and wives too." *Patrick, August 20, 2013.*